Anti-inflammatory Activity of Plant Polyphenols 2.0

Anti-inflammatory Activity of Plant Polyphenols 2.0

Editors

**Mario Dell'Agli
Enrico Sangiovanni**

MDPI • Basel • Beijing • Wuhan • Barcelona • Belgrade • Manchester • Tokyo • Cluj • Tianjin

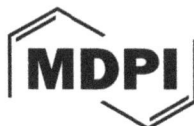

Editors
Mario Dell'Agli
Università degli Studi di Milano
Italy

Enrico Sangiovanni
Università degli Studi di Milano
Italy

Editorial Office
MDPI
St. Alban-Anlage 66
4052 Basel, Switzerland

This is a reprint of articles from the Special Issue published online in the open access journal *Biomedicines* (ISSN 2227-9059) (available at: https://www.mdpi.com/journal/biomedicines/special_issues/polyphenols_2).

For citation purposes, cite each article independently as indicated on the article page online and as indicated below:

LastName, A.A.; LastName, B.B.; LastName, C.C. Article Title. *Journal Name* **Year**, *Volume Number*, Page Range.

ISBN 978-3-0365-3196-0 (Hbk)
ISBN 978-3-0365-3197-7 (PDF)

© 2022 by the authors. Articles in this book are Open Access and distributed under the Creative Commons Attribution (CC BY) license, which allows users to download, copy and build upon published articles, as long as the author and publisher are properly credited, which ensures maximum dissemination and a wider impact of our publications.
The book as a whole is distributed by MDPI under the terms and conditions of the Creative Commons license CC BY-NC-ND.

Contents

About the Editors vii

Enrico Sangiovanni and Mario Dell'Agli
Special Issue: Anti-Inflammatory Activity of Plant Polyphenols 2.0
Reprinted from: *Biomedicines* **2021**, *10*, 37, doi:10.3390/biomedicines10010037 1

Shoib Sarwar Siddiqui, Sofia Rahman, H.P. Vasantha Rupasinghe and Cijo George Vazhappilly
Dietary Flavonoids in p53—Mediated Immune Dysfunctions Linking to Cancer Prevention
Reprinted from: *Biomedicines* **2020**, *8*, 286, doi:10.3390/biomedicines8080286 5

Alessandra Galli, Paola Marciani, Algerta Marku, Silvia Ghislanzoni, Federico Bertuzzi, Raffaella Rossi, Alessia Di Giancamillo, Michela Castagna and Carla Perego
Verbascoside Protects Pancreatic β-Cells against ER-Stress
Reprinted from: *Biomedicines* **2020**, *8*, 582, doi:10.3390/biomedicines8120582 37

Natalya N. Besednova, Boris G. Andryukov, Tatyana S. Zaporozhets, Sergey P. Kryzhanovsky, Ludmila N. Fedyanina, Tatyana A. Kuznetsova, Tatyana N. Zvyagintseva and Mikhail Yu. Shchelkanov
Antiviral Effects of Polyphenols from Marine Algae
Reprinted from: *Biomedicines* **2021**, *9*, 200, doi:10.3390/biomedicines9020200 53

Bryan Veeren, Matthieu Bringart, Chloe Turpin, Philippe Rondeau, Cynthia Planesse, Imade Ait-Arsa, Fanny Gimié, Claude Marodon, Olivier Meilhac, Marie-Paule Gonthier, Nicolas Diotel and Jean-Loup Bascands
Caffeic Acid, One of the Major Phenolic Acids of the Medicinal Plant *Antirhea borbonica*, Reduces Renal Tubulointerstitial Fibrosis
Reprinted from: *Biomedicines* **2021**, *9*, 358, doi:10.3390/biomedicines9040358 75

Vasiliki Zoi, Vasiliki Galani, Evrysthenis Vartholomatos, Natalia Żacharopoulou, Eftichia Tsoumeleka, Georgios Gkizas, Georgios Bozios, Pericles Tsekeris, Ieremias Chousidis, Ioannis Leonardos, Andreas G. Tzakos, Athanasios P. Kyritsis and George A. Alexiou
Curcumin and Radiotherapy Exert Synergistic Anti-Glioma Effect In Vitro
Reprinted from: *Biomedicines* **2021**, *9*, 1562, doi:10.3390/biomedicines9111562 97

About the Editors

Mario Dell'Agli is Full Professor in Pharmacognosy (2019-today) at the Department of Pharmacological and Biomolecular Sciences, Università degli Studi di Milano (Italy). He obtained a degree in Pharmaceutical Chemistry and Technology, Diploma of Specialty in Experimental Pharmacology, and Ph.D. in Pharmaco-toxicological, Pharmacognostical Sciences, and Pharmacological Biotechnologies. Mario Dell'Agli is currently the Head of the Laboratory of Pharmacognosy in Milan (2012-today). His research activity is devoted to the study of the biological and pharmacological activities of natural products derived from medicinal and edible plants. His research activity is documented by 90 peer reviewed papers (h-index: 28, Scopus). He is also a reviewer for more than 30 journals and an Editorial Board member/Editor for 5 international journals. He is co-author of more than 250 abstracts and scientific meetings and an invited speaker at 30 National and International meetings.

Enrico Sangiovanni is a Tenured Research Associate (RTD-B) at Department of Pharmacological and Biomolecular Sciences (DiSFeB) of Università degli Studi di Milano (UNIMI), where he investigates the anti-inflammatory activity of natural products at gastrointestinal and cutaneous level. In his career he has participated in six funded research projects and obtained funding as Principal Investigator for the study of the anti-inflammatory activities of *Cannabis sativa* L. and *Hamamelis virginiana* L. at a topical level. Dr. Sangiovanni has more than 70 contributions to Congresses, 54 international scientific publications, and is the author of 3 book chapters. Since 2011 he has been a member of the Interuniversity Center for Research on Malaria (CIRM) and since 2012 of the Italian Society of Pharmacology (SIF). Dr. Sangiovanni is member of the IUPHAR Mediterranean Group of Natural Products Pharmacology (IMGNPP) committee for the enhancement of natural products from the Mediterranean area.

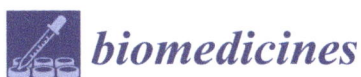

Editorial

Special Issue: Anti-Inflammatory Activity of Plant Polyphenols 2.0

Enrico Sangiovanni * and Mario Dell'Agli

Department of Pharmacological and Biomolecular Sciences, Università degli Studi di Milano, Via Balzaretti 9, 20133 Milano, Italy; mario.dellagli@unimi.it
* Correspondence: enrico.sangiovanni@unimi.it; Tel.: +39-02-5031-8383

Citation: Sangiovanni, E.; Dell'Agli, M. Special Issue: Anti-Inflammatory Activity of Plant Polyphenols 2.0. *Biomedicines* 2022, 10, 37. https://doi.org/10.3390/biomedicines10010037

Received: 20 December 2021
Accepted: 21 December 2021
Published: 24 December 2021

Publisher's Note: MDPI stays neutral with regard to jurisdictional claims in published maps and institutional affiliations.

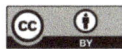

Copyright: © 2021 by the authors. Licensee MDPI, Basel, Switzerland. This article is an open access article distributed under the terms and conditions of the Creative Commons Attribution (CC BY) license (https://creativecommons.org/licenses/by/4.0/).

1. Introduction

Inflammation is a complex process that occurs in response to infections or other tissue damages, such as trauma, wounds, burns, and toxic substances. The inflammatory reaction is part of the human immune defense system and, macroscopically, can be characterized by five typical symptoms, mainly caused by local vascular changes and leukocyte activation: heat, redness, pain, swelling, and temporary loss of function. Overall, this fundamental process aims to protect the human body by avoiding the spread of harmful agents and to restore tissues and cellular homeostasis. However, when the causative agent is not properly removed, a chronic inflammatory state can occur.

Over time, the chronic stress causes damages ranging from loss of tissue function to DNA mutations, which can promote cancer cell formation. In this progression of damage, the continuous production of reactive oxygen species (ROS) plays a determining role. Oxidative stress is described as an altered equilibrium between the generation of ROS and the endogenous antioxidant defenses.

The plant kingdom remains an important resource of molecules with therapeutic potential for humans. Several plants have been shown to possess anti-inflammatory activities in clinical studies owing to the presence of secondary metabolites [1,2]. Polyphenols can directly act against pathogens such as viruses and bacteria, thus indirectly resolving the inflammatory process, as extensively demonstrated in propolis [3,4].

Nuclear factor κB (NF-κB) is a key transcription factor responsible for the expression of cytokines, chemokines, and other cellular inflammatory mediators and is considered one of the main proinflammatory pathways [5]. In physiological conditions, this factor is found in an inactive form in the cytoplasm, bound to its own inhibitory protein IκBα. However, the presence of proinflammatory stimuli, such as infections, ROS, or other endogenous proinflammatory mediators, leads to the rapid activation of NF-κB, which translocates into the nucleus. NF-κB is an excellent target for evaluating the anti-inflammatory activity of various molecules, including those of plant origin. In fact, several classes of polyphenols can inhibit the action of this transcription factor in different cellular models [6–8].

Polyphenols are molecules with excellent antioxidant capacity owing to the presence of phenolic rings, which act as electron traps for ROS. Despite this direct action, the most recent scientific evidence has shown that the best antioxidant activity is obtained by the stimulation of endogenous antioxidant defenses.

Nuclear factor erythroid 2–related factor 2 (Nrf2) regulates the expression of endogenous antioxidant enzymes, such as catalase and superoxide dismutase. In resting conditions, this factor is bound to its inhibitory protein, the kelch-like ECH associated protein (Keap1). Nrf2 is activated by increased oxidative stress, which induces the detachment from Keap1 and the binding of Nrf2 to the antioxidant element (ARE), hence promoting the transcription of cytoprotective enzymes [9].

Oxidative stress plays a dual role in inflamed cells; on the one hand, it is a fundamental factor for signal transmission for immunomodulation and apoptosis, but on the other hand, it is a potential source of DNA mutations, capable of inducing DNA strand lesions and nitration of the guanine bases. Between the several genes implicated in DNA damages and repair response, the tumor suppressor p53 gene has a key role, acting as a transcription regulator under stress conditions.

The NF-κB, Nrf2, and p53 pathways are deeply connected, and their regulation can change the cellular fate. For example, p53 acts as a suppressor of inflammation, and it can inhibit the transcriptional activity of NF-κB [10].

The purpose of this Special Issue is to contribute to the collection of scientific evidence on the anti-inflammatory properties of polyphenols, focusing on the role of individual compounds and their respective mechanisms of action, including anti-inflammatory and antioxidant effects.

2. Recent Advances in the Role of Polyphenols in Inflammatory Conditions

In this Special Issue, scientific papers concerning different pathological contexts are collected, from renal function to antiviral properties, but also cancer prevention. The studies include both in vitro and in vivo effects and describe bioavailability data of active principles, when available. This collection focuses mainly on pure compounds and the mechanisms of action underlying their anti-inflammatory and antioxidant activities.

Galli A. et al. [11] investigated the effect of verbascoside on pancreatic β-cells. This phenylethanoid glycoside is present in the wastewater of olive fruit processing. Verbascoside can be extracted from *Olea europea*, but also from other plant families. The authors demonstrated that verbascoside prevents β-cells' oxidative stress by decreasing ROS content and lipid peroxidation through the activation of the Nrf2 pathway. In addition, verbascoside reduced the activation of the NF-κB pathway, protecting pancreatic β-cells from death, but also preserved the mitochondrial membrane potential under basal and stressed conditions. These effects were obtained by treating cells with a concentration of 16 μM of verbascoside. The results of this study set the basis for the possible use of verbascoside in protecting β-cells from oxidative stress and inflammation, conditions involved in type 2 diabetes progression.

Curcumin is a well-known curcuminoid extracted from the rhizome of *Curcuma longa*. Various biological activities of curcumin have been described in the literature including antioxidant, antimicrobial, and anti-inflammatory properties [12]. Zoi V. et al. [13] explored the possible use of curcumin as a radio-sensitizing agent in the treatment of glioblastoma, the most common and severe malignant brain tumor. The authors discovered that curcumin (3–26 μM) improves the radiosensitive status of glioblastoma cancer cells (U87 and T98, exposed to 2 Gy or 4 Gy of irradiation), resulting in a higher inhibitory effect compared to radiation or curcumin alone. The mechanism of action involved G2/M arrest in the cell cycle. Furthermore, curcumin showed synergistic effects even when combined with the chemotherapeutic agent temozolomide. Other researchers have positively described the association of curcumin with other chemotherapeutic agents [14] and the use of liposomal formulations [15]. These findings encourage further studies to evaluate the potential use of curcumin alongside radiotherapy as an innovative strategy for the treatment of glioblastoma.

Vereen B. et al. evaluated the anti-renal fibrosis effect of an extract from *Antirhea borbonica*, a French medicinal plant found in Reunion Island, in comparison to caffeic acid, one of the major phenolic acids of the extract, in mice subjected to unilateral ureteral obstruction [16]. Mice were treated daily with an oral dose of 25 mg/kg of *Antirhea borbonica* or 25 mg/kg of caffeic acid by gavage. Both the extract and caffeic acid reduced macrophage infiltration and induced a down-regulation of pro-inflammatory and pro-fibrotic cytokines (Tgf-β, Tnf-α), chemokines (Mcp1), and inhibition of NF-κB. Polyphenols from *Antirhea borbonica* also significantly increased Nrf2 mRNA expression and subsequent CAT and Cu/ZnSOD enzymes. The authors concluded that the in vivo nephroprotective effects of *Antirhea borbonica* is partially supported by the presence of caffeic acid, but the contribution of other polyphenols present in the plant extract cannot be excluded.

Siddiqui S.S. et al. reviewed the effects of the main dietary flavonoids focusing on their ability to prevent inflammation and cancer in relation to p53-mediated mechanisms [17]. The flavonoids explored by the authors were quercetin, luteolin, cyanidin, daidzein, and epigallocatechin gallate (EGCG). This group of flavonoids exert their anti-inflammatory effects mainly by inhibiting the Janus kinase-signal transducer and activator of transcription (JAK-STAT), NF-κB, and mitogen-activated protein kinase (MAPK) pathways. The effects involved a reduction in cytokines (IL-1β, TNF-α, IL-6, and IL-8) and cell death markers (caspase-3). The authors concluded that these flavonoids could reduce inflammation and ultimately lead to cancer prevention, thus emphasizing the need for further studies to explore the connections between the p53 and Nrf2 pathways.

Finally, the study of Besdnova N.N. considered the antiviral effects of polyphenols from marine algae, reviewing the biological activities and their mechanism of actions [18]. Macro- and microalgae can accumulate phloroglucinol and related polymers, named phlorotannins. Phlorotannins are a class of heterogenous compounds in terms of molecular weight and level of isomerization; some of these structures can be sulphated or halogenated. Seaweed phlorotannins are composed of eight phenolic rings, which give a greater antioxidant power than that of tannins produced by terrestrial plants, which possess only three or four phenolic rings. The authors highlighted the ability of phlorotannins to decrease viral load, acting at different stages of the viral cell cycle by interfering, for example, with the attachment to the cell surface, exerting a direct antiviral effect or blocking viral enzymes. Concomitantly, phlorotannins can enhance antioxidant defense and reduce inflammation by lowering the production of proinflammatory cytokines and inflammatory cell migration.

3. Conclusions and Future Perspectives

The data collected in this Special Issue once again confirm the importance of the plant kingdom for the search for new compounds with anti-inflammatory activity. Inflammation plays a central role in various pathological contexts, ranging from acute infection to metabolic or chronic damages. The scientific literature underlines the close correlation between inflammatory markers, ROS, and DNA damage; the latter is capable of increasing the probability of tumor formations.

In this context, polyphenols can play a fundamental role both in curative and preventive terms, also due to their dietary intake. Despite the large body of preclinical literature, there is still a lack of clinical data on polyphenols that can confirm their activities in humans, especially in the case of extracts intended as mixtures of different components. The main limitations are due to the variability of the composition of the plant matrices and the lack of titration in active ingredients. However, these studies confirm that even isolated polyphenols can have interesting biological activities.

Although polyphenols have shown various benefits in the inflammatory field, one of the main limitations for their use in humans concerns their bioavailability. In this regard, various strategies are being studied to improve the absorption of these compounds, and the use of phytosomal formulations appears to be one of the most promising ways [19].

Funding: This research received no external funding.

Institutional Review Board Statement: Not applicable.

Informed Consent Statement: Not applicable.

Conflicts of Interest: The authors declare no conflict of interest.

References

1. Di Lorenzo, C.; Dell'agli, M.; Badea, M.; Dima, L.; Colombo, E.; Sangiovanni, E.; Restani, P.; Bosisio, E. Plant Food Supplements with Anti-Inflammatory Properties: A Systematic Review (II). *Crit. Rev. Food Sci. Nutr.* **2013**, *53*, 507–516. [CrossRef] [PubMed]
2. Dell'Agli, M.; Di Lorenzo, C.; Badea, M.; Sangiovanni, E.; Dima, L.; Bosisio, E.; Restani, P. Plant food supplements with anti-inflammatory properties: A systematic review (I). *Crit. Rev. Food Sci. Nutr.* **2013**, *53*, 403–413. [CrossRef] [PubMed]
3. Magnavacca, A.; Sangiovanni, E.; Racagni, G.; Dell'Agli, M. The antiviral and immunomodulatory activities of propolis: An update and future perspectives for respiratory diseases. *Med. Res. Rev.* **2021**. Online ahead of print. [CrossRef] [PubMed]

4. Przybylek, I.; Karpinski, T.M. Antibacterial Properties of Propolis. *Molecules* **2019**, *24*, 2047. [CrossRef] [PubMed]
5. Lawrence, T. The nuclear factor NF-kappaB pathway in inflammation. *Cold Spring Harb. Perspect. Biol.* **2009**, *1*, a001651. [CrossRef] [PubMed]
6. Magnavacca, A.; Piazza, S.; Cammisa, A.; Fumagalli, M.; Martinelli, G.; Giavarini, F.; Sangiovanni, E.; Dell'Agli, M. Ribes nigrum Leaf Extract Preferentially Inhibits IFN-gamma-Mediated Inflammation in HaCaT Keratinocytes. *Molecules* **2021**, *26*, 3044. [CrossRef] [PubMed]
7. Nwakiban, A.P.A.; Fumagalli, M.; Piazza, S.; Magnavacca, A.; Martinelli, G.; Beretta, G.; Magni, P.; Tchamgoue, A.D.; Agbor, G.A.; Kuiate, J.R.; et al. Dietary Cameroonian Plants Exhibit Anti-Inflammatory Activity in Human Gastric Epithelial Cells. *Nutrients* **2020**, *12*, 3787. [CrossRef] [PubMed]
8. Piazza, S.; Pacchetti, B.; Fumagalli, M.; Bonacina, F.; Dell'Agli, M.; Sangiovanni, E. Comparison of Two Ginkgo biloba L. Extracts on Oxidative Stress and Inflammation Markers in Human Endothelial Cells. *Mediat. Inflamm.* **2019**, *2019*, 6173893. [CrossRef]
9. Baird, L.; Yamamoto, M. The Molecular Mechanisms Regulating the KEAP1-NRF2 Pathway. *Mol. Cell. Biol.* **2020**, *40*, e00099-20. [CrossRef]
10. Barabutis, N.; Schally, A.V.; Siejka, A. P53, GHRH, inflammation and cancer. *EBioMedicine* **2018**, *37*, 557–562. [CrossRef]
11. Galli, A.; Marciani, P.; Marku, A.; Ghislanzoni, S.; Bertuzzi, F.; Rossi, R.; Di Giancamillo, A.; Castagna, M.; Perego, C. Verbascoside Protects Pancreatic beta-Cells against ER-Stress. *Biomedicines* **2020**, *8*, 582. [CrossRef] [PubMed]
12. Canistro, D.; Chiavaroli, A.; Cicia, D.; Cimino, F.; Currò, D.; Dell'Agli, M.; Ferrante, C.; Giovannelli, L.; Leone, S.; Martinelli, G.; et al. The pharmacological basis of the curcumin nutraceutical uses: An update. *Pharmadvances* **2021**, *3*, 421–466. [CrossRef]
13. Zoi, V.; Galani, V.; Vartholomatos, E.; Zacharopoulou, N.; Tsoumeleka, E.; Gkizas, G.; Bozios, G.; Tsekeris, P.; Chousidis, I.; Leonardos, I.; et al. Curcumin and Radiotherapy Exert Synergistic Anti-Glioma Effect In Vitro. *Biomedicines* **2021**, *9*, 1562. [CrossRef] [PubMed]
14. Giordano, A.; Tommonaro, G. Curcumin and Cancer. *Nutrients* **2019**, *11*, 2376. [CrossRef] [PubMed]
15. Feng, T.; Wei, Y.; Lee, R.J.; Zhao, L. Liposomal curcumin and its application in cancer. *Int. J. Nanomed.* **2017**, *12*, 6027–6044. [CrossRef] [PubMed]
16. Veeren, B.; Bringart, M.; Turpin, C.; Rondeau, P.; Planesse, C.; Ait-Arsa, I.; Gimie, F.; Marodon, C.; Meilhac, O.; Gonthier, M.P.; et al. Caffeic Acid, One of the Major Phenolic Acids of the Medicinal Plant Antirhea borbonica, Reduces Renal Tubulointerstitial Fibrosis. *Biomedicines* **2021**, *9*, 358. [CrossRef] [PubMed]
17. Siddiqui, S.S.; Rahman, S.; Rupasinghe, H.P.V.; Vazhappilly, C.G. Dietary Flavonoids in p53-Mediated Immune Dysfunctions Linking to Cancer Prevention. *Biomedicines* **2020**, *8*, 286. [CrossRef] [PubMed]
18. Besednova, N.N.; Andryukov, B.G.; Zaporozhets, T.S.; Kryzhanovsky, S.P.; Fedyanina, L.N.; Kuznetsova, T.A.; Zvyagintseva, T.N.; Shchelkanov, M.Y. Antiviral Effects of Polyphenols from Marine Algae. *Biomedicines* **2021**, *9*, 200. [CrossRef] [PubMed]
19. Barani, M.; Sangiovanni, E.; Angarano, M.; Rajizadeh, M.A.; Mehrabani, M.; Piazza, S.; Gangadharappa, H.V.; Pardakhty, A.; Mehrbani, M.; Dell'Agli, M.; et al. Phytosomes as Innovative Delivery Systems for Phytochemicals: A Comprehensive Review of Literature. *Int. J. Nanomed.* **2021**, *16*, 6983–7022. [CrossRef] [PubMed]

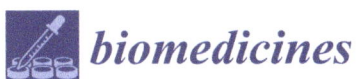 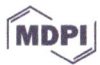

Review

Dietary Flavonoids in p53—Mediated Immune Dysfunctions Linking to Cancer Prevention

Shoib Sarwar Siddiqui [1], Sofia Rahman [2], H.P. Vasantha Rupasinghe [3,4] and Cijo George Vazhappilly [1,*]

[1] Department of Biotechnology, American University of Ras Al Khaimah, Ras Al Khaimah PO Box 10021, UAE; shoib.siddiqui@aurak.ac.ae
[2] School of Natural Sciences and Mathematics, The University of Texas at Dallas, Richardson, TX 75080, USA; sofiarahman0@gmail.com
[3] Department of Plant, Food, and Environmental Sciences, Faculty of Agriculture, Dalhousie University, Truro, NS B2N 5E3, Canada; vrupasinghe@dal.ca
[4] Department of Pathology, Faculty of Medicine, Dalhousie University, Halifax, NS B3H 4R2, Canada
* Correspondence: cijo.vazhappilly@aurak.ac.ae

Received: 29 June 2020; Accepted: 11 August 2020; Published: 13 August 2020

Abstract: The p53 protein plays a central role in mediating immune functioning and determines the fate of the cells. Its role as a tumor suppressor, and in transcriptional regulation and cytokine activity under stress conditions, is well defined. The wild type (WT) p53 functions as a guardian for the genome, while the mutant p53 has oncogenic roles. One of the ways that p53 combats carcinogenesis is by reducing inflammation. WT p53 functions as an anti-inflammatory molecule via cross-talk activity with multiple immunological pathways, such as the major histocompatibility complex I (MHCI) associated pathway, toll-like receptors (TLRs), and immune checkpoints. Due to the multifarious roles of p53 in cancer, it is a potent target for cancer immunotherapy. Plant flavonoids have been gaining recognition over the last two decades to use as a potential therapeutic regimen in ameliorating diseases. Recent studies have shown the ability of flavonoids to suppress chronic inflammation, specifically by modulating p53 responses. Further, the anti-oxidant Keap1/Nrf2/ARE pathway could play a crucial role in mitigating oxidative stress, leading to a reduction of chronic inflammation linked to the prevention of cancer. This review aims to discuss the pharmacological properties of plant flavonoids in response to various oxidative stresses and immune dysfunctions and analyzes the cross-talk between flavonoid-rich dietary intake for potential disease prevention.

Keywords: flavonoids; inflammation; p53; cancer prevention; Nrf2 pathway; anti-oxidant

---

1. Introduction

One of the hallmarks of cancer is genome instability due to DNA damage [1]. There are several genes implicated in modulating the pathways related to DNA damage and repair response [2]. An impetus to this field of research was provided by the discovery of the first tumor suppressor gene p53 in SV-transformed cells in 1979 [3]. However, the history of p53 is rather interesting. Initially, it was observed that p53 could accumulate in cancer cells and a knockdown of the gene led to the inhibition of cell proliferation. Thus, scientists presumed that it was an "oncogene." The identification of new oncogenes was fascinating [4]. However, over the last four decades, p53 has evolved from the realization of a tumor suppressor protein to transcription factor, a regulator of metabolic pathways, a regulator of cytokine activity, and a drug target for cancer therapy [4]. Due to its role in the DNA damage and repair process, the tumor suppressor *p53* gene is often referred to as the "guardian of the genome" [5].

Several reports and observations showed the role of p53 as an oncogene. However, it was observed in many tumor models that the mouse *Trp53* is inactivated by the retroviral insertions pointing towards its potential role as a tumor suppressor gene [6,7]. This p53 conundrum took a turn when the cloned wild type (WT) p53 sequence was compared with the tumor expressing p53 and it was observed that the tumor-promoting activity of p53 is due to its mutant form found in cancer cells [4]. In an elegant study on colorectal cancer, it was shown that more than 50% of tumors had a loss of heterozygosity (LOH) at the p53 locus, thus providing further evidence of its role as a tumor suppressor [8]. Further experiments strengthen the notion that the wild type p53 can suppress oncogenic transformation [9]. The analysis of p53 knockout mice was interesting. The mice were developmentally normal but developed primary lymphomas and sarcomas at around 6 to 9 months of age [10]. In human patients, the early clues came in the 1960s from the group of people who were highly prone to develop cancer due to a rare autosomal mutation. This syndrome was called Li-Fraumeni syndrome (LFS) [11,12]. Later, the specific mutation was identified as a germline mutation in *TP53* [13,14].

1.1. p53 as a Transcription Factor

p53 acts as a transcription regulator under stress conditions. After the acceptance of p53 as a tumor suppressor, several studies were published in the early 1990s leading to the role of p53 as a transcription factor [15–17]. Wild type p53 has been shown to have DNA binding ability, while its mutant counterpart, often found in cancer cells, does not have this ability [15–17]. Moreover, the effect of p53 as a transcription activator is direct, but the effect as a repressor is indirect [15–17]. Further, p53 regulates the transcription of genes that are important for apoptosis, cell cycle, and DNA repair machinery [4]. p53 functions as a pioneer transcription factor. The binding of p53 to nucleosomal DNA takes place through the linker DNAs. p53 also binds to histone protein through the N-terminal 1–93 amino acid region [18]. In a recent study, it was identified that the transcriptional regulation of porcine p53 is very similar to human p53 for a number of target genes, and, thus, it is inferred that pigs can be used to study human diseases [19]. The role of p53 as a transcription factor is also shown in several disease models. Human dihydroorotate dehydrogenase (DHODH) is an enzyme involved in de novo synthesis of pyrimidines. Tetrahydroindazoles (HZ) have been identified as potent inhibitors of DHODH. HZ analogs have been shown as promising agents against cancer progression. The cell-based reporter showed that HZ functions by activating the p53-dependent transcription activity [20]. The autosomal dominant polycystic kidney disease (ADPKD) is mainly caused by the mutations in the PKD1 or PKD2 genes. The recent studies showed that PKD1 gene expression is controlled by the overlapping but opposing transcriptional activity of Myc and p53 [21]. Esophageal Cancer-Related Gene 2 (ECRG2) is a tumor suppressor whose activity is highly regulated by the transcriptional activity of p53. It was identified for two p53 binding sites within the promoter of ECRG2, and thus its mRNA and protein expression is regulated [22].

1.2. p53 as a Regulator of Metabolic Pathways

One of the hallmarks of cancer is the shift to glycolysis as the predominant metabolic pathway for the generation of energy, despite oxidative phosphorylation being an efficient way to produce adenosine triphosphate (ATP). This is referred to as the "Warburg effect." Due to this, cancer cells utilize a higher amount of glucose compared to normal cells. Both the oncogenes and tumor suppressor genes have been shown to play a pivotal role in the regulation of this phenomenon. p53 is one of the factors that reduce the utilization of glycolysis and enhance the oxidative phosphorylation of cancer cells [23]. Thus, p53 plays a vital role in this metabolic pathway, which is also a hallmark for cancer cells [1]. p53, together with other tumor suppressor genes, carries out the function of immunological homeostasis. Moreover, the transcriptional activity of p53 regulates the expression and signaling of a number of cytokines and some of these cytokines activate p53 expression suggesting a positive feedback loop. In addition, the immune checkpoint regulators, such as program cell death protein 1

(PD1) and program cell death ligand 1 (PDL1), also cross-talk with p53 and thus modulate the overall immune responses [24].

1.3. p53 as a Drug Target for Cancer

As discussed previously, more than 50% of all cancer has a p53 mutation [25]. p53 is important for homeostatic signaling in cell proliferation, cell cycle regulation, apoptosis, senescence, and inflammation, and a mutation in this crucial protein leads to malignancy. The most common mutation in p53 is a single amino acid substitution, which leads to the loss of DNA binding function and misfolding of the protein. There has been a thrust to develop drugs that can restore the WT activity in the missense mutant proteins. This restoration of WT activity in mutant p53 is often referred to as a "reactivating mutant" [26]. Although many such drug candidates have been developed, most of them failed during the early developmental phase [26]. The reactivation of p53 is a major pharmacological intervention and has been suggested to have promising effects for cancer therapy. PhiKan083, also known as PK083, has been shown to reactivate p53 mutants under pre-clinical settings. Using virtual screening and validation on different p53 mutants, it was shown that Y220C and Y220S are the targets of PK083 [27]. In another study with virtual screening on natural compounds targeting the Loop1/Sheet 3 (L1/S3) of WT-p53, a drug candidate torilin was identified. Torilin not only improved p53 activity but also enhanced protein expression of p21. This ultimately led to the suppression of HCT116 cancer cell growth [28]. It is noteworthy that around 80% of triple-negative breast cancer (TNBC) patients have a mutation in p53. Therefore, reactivating p53 mutants by drugs can be prolific for clinical intervention. One such drug recently studied for TNBC is 2-sulfonylpyrimidine compound, PK11007. PK11007 targets the apoptotic pathway of cell death in TNBC cell lines [29]. These recent studies highlighted the role of p53 as an attractive drug target for cancer therapy.

2. p53-Mediated Inflammatory Response and Immune Signaling

The role of inflammation in the promotion of cancer is well defined and is considered as an important hallmark of the disease [1]. Cancer leads to inflammation and in many instances, chronic inflammation leads to cancer [30]. The oxidative stress induced by reactive oxygen and nitrogen species [31] and viral and bacterial infection is associated with cancer risk [32]. How p53 is involved in cancer-related inflammation in the tumor microenvironment is an interesting question. p53 acts as a suppressor of inflammation, but proof came from the p53 knockout mouse, which itself led to chronic inflammation in mice, but not sufficient enough to cause cancer. It was observed that many of the mice died before the progression of the tumor due to chronic inflammation [10,33]. In an experimental autoimmune encephalomyelitis (EAE) model, p53 knockout mice showed severe inflammation in the central nervous system (CNS) [34]. In a collagen-induced arthritis (CIA) model, p53 knock out mice developed more severe arthritis symptoms compared to WT DBA/1 mice [35]. This is further proof for the role of p53 as an anti-inflammatory target. Using an azoxymethane (AOM)-induced colon cancer model in a conditional knockout mouse of p53, it was shown that the loss of p53 in stem cells leads to tumor formation with a combinational effect of DNA damage and chronic inflammation [36].

Further, to identify the functioning of p53 as an anti-inflammatory agent, several studies have been carried out and linked with the transcription factor nuclear factor-κB (NF-κB). p53 suppresses the activity of NF-κB by inhibiting the transcriptional activity of p65 or suppressing the activation of p65 by IκB kinase (IKK) and proteasomal degradation of IκB. It is noteworthy that IκB acts as an inhibitor of NF-κB [37,38]. In the studies pertaining to gastric cancer caused by *Helicobacter Pylori*, it has been shown that the virulence factor cytotoxin-associated gene A (CagA) activates NF-κB and induces inflammation in gastric epithelial cells [39–41]. This activation of NF-κB further enhances the expression of activation-induced cytidine deaminase (AICDA), which promotes cancer by incorporating *TP53* mutations [42]. In addition, the inflammatory bowel diseases are characterized by the infiltration of neutrophils that are rich sources of free radical species. These free radicals have been shown to promote cancer progression by incorporating mutations in the *TP53* gene [39,43,44].

2.1. Cross-Talk between p53 and MHCI Pathway

The major histocompatibility complex (MHC), derived the name from its discovery with the research on tissue compatibility upon transplantation. These are an important class of gene complexes that play a pivotal role in recognition of foreign antigens. Being expressed on the cell surface, they interact with T-cell receptors (TCR) and pose an immune response against the endogenous or exogenous antigens [45]. MHCI is expressed on the surface of all nucleated cells (epithelial or fibroblasts) and is involved in showcasing the intracellular proteins on the cell surface in the form of short peptides. The processing and transport of these small peptides is a complex process that involves the interplay of several proteins, including transporter associated with antigen processing 1 (TAP1) and TAP2. It has been shown previously that one of the alleles of MHCI, human leukocyte antigen B7, can be transcriptionally repressed by the tumor suppressor gene p53 [46]. Several other studies pointed out that p53 can promote the processing of peptides inside the cell and modulate the surface expression of MHC1 [47,48]. In addition to these changes, the transcriptional activity of p53 can upregulate the expression of TAP1 (a protein involved in the transport of peptides toMHC1).

Moreover, p53 also upregulates the expression of ERAP1 (endoplasmic reticulum aminopeptidase 1), which leads to enhanced expression of MHCI on the cell surface [47,48]. The cumulative effect of this p53 processing resulted in an enhanced immune response against cancer. Interestingly, the mutant p53 has lost the activity of all these processes, which emphasizes the dysregulated immune function and oncogenic role of mutant p53. On the contrary, it has been observed that the loss of function of important genes in the MHCI processing pathway, such as β2 microglobulin and TAP1, also leads to a reduction in the function of p53, proposing a cross-talk between MHCI and the p53 pathway [39]. In a recent study, it was shown that the lack of p53 in medulloblastoma leads to the loss of MHCI expression and resistance to immune rejection. The mechanistic study showed that this is due to the loss of expression of TAP1 and ERAP1, but tumor necrosis factor factor-alpha (TNF-α) agonists can rescue the expression of these proteins. Moreover, in vivo studies also supported the notion that the p53 null state plays a pivotal role in immune evasion, and TNF can reverse this phenotype [49].

2.2. Cross-Talk between p53 and Immune Checkpoints

To mount an immune response, the MHCI showcase the peptide to the surface of the TCR of T cells. Once activated, T cells start to express PD1 that react with PD-L1. This PD1/PDL1 axis is instrumental in maintaining the protective immunity and homeostatic condition. Beside PD1/PDL1, a flurry of other receptor–ligand complexes keep the immune system in check. These receptor–ligand complexes are called immune checkpoints [50]. These immune checkpoints are vital for maintaining the physiological resting state of immune cells (T cells). However, in the case of cancer progression, cancer cells hijack this process and engage T cells for immune evasion. The overexpression of PDL1 ligands on their surface of cancer cells to engage with PD1 of T cells is well recognized. This engagement of PD1 with PDL1 ultimately leads to immunosuppression [51]. Targeting this pathway is considered as a hotspot for cancer immunotherapy. It was identified that miR-34a, which acts as a transcriptional target of p53, is actually a repressor of PDL1. Thus, p53/miR-34a/PDL1 can be a suitable target for cancer immunotherapy [52]. A loss of p53 activity by a mutation in human lung cancer has been shown to upregulate PD-L1 expression. Thus it will be instrumental in predicting the patient pool that may or may not be responsive to checkpoint inhibitors targeting the PD1/PDL1 axis [53].

2.3. Cross-Talk between p53 and TLRs

Toll-like receptors (TLRs) are the receptors that detect pathogen-associated molecular patterns (PAMPs), present mostly on the microbial surfaces [54]. Many TLRs were also found on the surface of cancer cells as well. TLR signaling on cancer cells mediates a number of functions that trigger cancer progression. Therefore, TLRs are considered as another attractive target for cancer immunotherapy [55]. It was shown that p53 could act as a transcriptional activator of TLR3 that can trigger agonist-induced apoptosis in cancer cells [56]. There is a cross-talk between the target genes of p53 and TLRs, and they together mediate the downstream signaling [57]. In the patients with mutant p53, the TLR4 expression inversely correlates with the survival time, and in the WT p53 patients, the TLR4 expression correlates directly with the survival time [58]. TLR8 is a target of p53 where its expression was increased due to a single nucleotide polymorphism (SNP) (rs3761624) in the TLR8 promoter [59]. In another study, a comparison of the expression of TLR1-TLR10, p53, and NF-κB in patients of oral lichenoid disease (OLD) with healthy individuals was interpreted. It was found that all TLRs and p53 were increased in OLD versus healthy individuals in all the layers. Moreover, a positive correlation was obtained between the expression of TLR5, NF-κB, and p53 in the intermediate layer in OLD patients [60]. Thus, there is a cross-talk between TLRs and p53 in the pathology of OLD. TLR4 is important in vascular inflammation, atherosclerosis, and diabetes. In the study to identify the role of palmitate-triggered apoptosis in the activation of TLR4 associated pathways, it was found that the palmitate promoted apoptosis in vascular smooth muscle cells (VSMC) and significantly enhanced the expression of p53. The knockdown of TLR4 led to a reduction in the expression of p53 in this model, directing towards the role of the TLR4/p53 axis in atherosclerosis [61]. Further, imiquimod (IMQ) is a synthetic TLR7 ligand used for the treatment of basal cell carcinoma (BCC). A thorough study was carried out in order to understand the role of p53 in IMQ triggered cell death in the skin cancer model. It was identified that IMQ could lead to the upregulation of p53 expression, its phosphorylation, and translocation in a TLR7/8-independent manner [62].

3. p53 in the Tumor Microenvironment and Cancer Immunotherapy

The tumor microenvironment is very important in determining the fate of the tumor and its progression. One of the factors that shape the tumor microenvironment is p53. It has recently been shown that a loss of p53 can dramatically affect the immune cell composition of tumors [63,64] (Figure 1). The tumor-promoting macrophages are recruited in breast cancer, prostate cancer, and ovarian cancer with the loss of p53 [63–65]. On the other hand, p53 loss increases the response of tumor-associated macrophages (TAMs) to a variety of tumor types such as lung, pancreatic, ovarian, and carcinogen-induced skin cancers [65,66]. In the breast cancer model, the loss of p53 has been shown to involve the malfunctioning of the WNT pathway and infiltration of neutrophils, which supports cancer progression [63]. The infiltration of monocytes in the ascites of ovarian cancer is observed in p53 null state, probably due to the involvement of the C-C motif chemokine ligand 2 (CCL2) [65]. In p53 null tumors, the infiltration of tumor-suppressive myeloid CD11b$^+$ cells and Treg was observed. The expression of C-C chemokine receptor type 2 (CCR2) associated chemokine and macrophage colony-stimulating factor (M-CSF) were responsible for blunting the immune response by targeting T helper and T cytotoxic cells [67]. Thus, tumor cells get the advantage of manipulating the immune microenvironment by the loss of p53 or the accumulation of mutations in p53 [39].

p53 as a Target for Cancer Immunotherapy

Since p53 is highly regarded as a mutated gene in tumors, it can act as a target for cancer immunotherapy. Due to the intracellular localization of p53, targeting through antibodies was not possible. However, in a recent study, a novel antibody T1-116C was generated, which acts as a TCR mimic. This antibody recognizes several cancer types without recognizing normal blood cells. In the breast cancer xenograft model, it was showed to significantly reduce tumor growth [68]. A similar approach with affinity matured human antibody, P1C1TM, was shown to be effective in reducing the tumor growth both in vitro and in vivo [69]. In a recent report, the role of p53 in systemic inflammation was deciphered. In the breast cancer models, a loss of p53 in cancer cells led to an increase in WNT ligands, which triggered the macrophages to produce interleukin 1 beta (IL-1β) that ultimately led to systemic inflammation. Thus, this study was a direct demonstration of p53 as a mediator of inflammation, neutrophilia, and metastasis [63].

Constitutive activation of the signal transducer and activator of transcription 3 (STAT3) pathway is an important factor in determining the tumor stroma and hence considered as a potential target for cancer immunotherapy [70]. It is known that the loss of p53 leads to constitutive activation of the STAT3 pathway in pancreatic cancer. Moreover, the mutations in *p53* genes in human pancreatic cancer correlate with the poor prognosis and survival time [71]. In addition, the ablation of p53 also leads to enhanced reactive oxygen species (ROS) production that inhibits Src homology region 2 (SHP2) activation and triggers STAT3 expression [71]. In a phosphatase and tensin homolog (PTEN) knockout mouse and embryonic fibroblasts, p53 deficiency led to an increase in STAT3-myc signaling [72]. STAT3 is negatively regulated by suppressors of cytokine signaling 1 (SOCS1) protein that binds to the N-terminal domain of p53, leading to cell cycle arrest and senescence [73]. One of the mutants of p53, R175H, has been shown to enhance NF-κB signaling and increased localization to one of its subunits p65 [74]. Some of the mutants of p53 proteins also directly interact with p65 leading to increasing NF-κB transcriptional activity [75]. It has shown that the mutant p53 protein inhibits the expression of secreted interleukin-1 receptor antagonist (sIL-1Ra) and, thus, promotes malignancy. sIL-1Ra is a target gene for mutp53 and thus, a potential therapeutic target for combating tumor growth [76]. *TP53* gene mutation is frequent in hepatocellular carcinoma (HCC). As discussed earlier, p53/mir-34a/PD-L1 and TLRs can also be considered as targets for cancer immunotherapy.

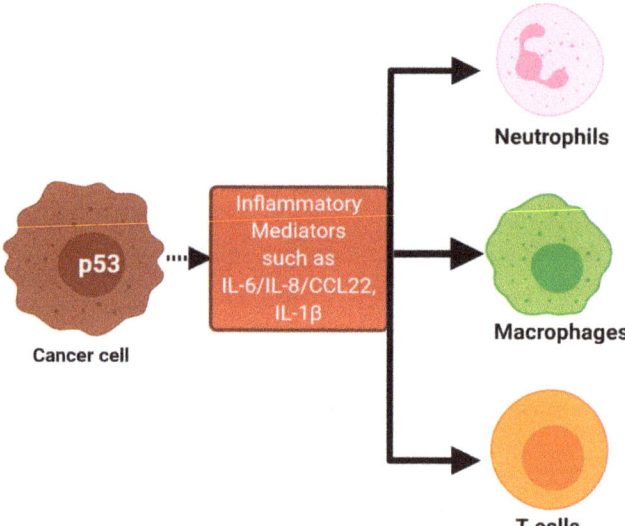

Figure 1. Infiltration of immune cells due to activation of p53: The activation of p53 in cancer cells can be due to many factors such as TLR5-flagellin interaction. Due to this activation of p53, the inflammatory mediators are released, which leads to the infiltration of immune cells in the tumor microenvironment. These immune cells include neutrophils, macrophages, and T cells.

4. Chronic Inflammation and Cancer

Invasion of pathogens, increased toxicity in the cells, or tissue injuries are some of the traumas that the human body combats with the progression of inflammation. Activation of inflammation is initiated by immune cells such as mast cells and macrophages, and progressively results in the production of inflammatory mediators, such as pro-inflammatory cytokines and chemokines, whose roles are to amplify the inflammatory response in order to resolve the trauma [77]. Collectively, these inflammatory reactions lead to the release of ROS and reactive nitrogen species (RNS), in attempts to aim for tissue repairing by cellular and immune changes concluding in the amendments of the site of injured cells by cell proliferation [78]. Thus, it can be noted that the purpose of inflammation is to solve the cellular impairments and restore cellular homeostasis. Similar to every homeostatic maintenance behavior, the initial process should be able to shut down after the resolution of the initiator. Therefore, in this case, after the restoration of the damaged tissue by the regular rate of cell growth, the inflammatory processes should be able to suspend and establish inflammation resolution through multiple mechanisms. One for instance, is moving from pro-inflammatory to anti-inflammatory reactions by the intervention of the released ROS [79]. However, if the ability of the inflammation is not resolvable, it results in the building up of the inflammatory response products, and transformation from acute inflammation to prolonged chronic inflammation. Another source of chronic inflammation has been identified as when the acute inflammatory processes are unable to rectify the cellular damages, thus becoming uncontrolled and chronic, which further play a role in the development of chronic inflammatory diseases [80]. In chronic inflammation, the immune cells maintain a pro-inflammatory nature, aggravating the by-products released by the immune cells, which co-results in continuous uncontrolled cell proliferation. ROS and RNS are two such by-products that are considered to aid in chronic inflammation-related cancer [81]. Additionally, ROS and RNS are sources of DNA mutations, as they generate peroxynitrite. Peroxynitrite has been defined to possess mutagenic properties such as DNA strand lesions and nitration of the guanine bases [82]. The 8-oxo-7,8-dihydro-2′-deoxyguanosine (8-oxodG) and 8-nitroguanine are the examples of the DNA breakages formed by the ROS and RNS, which are known to exhibit DNA mutations and have been indicated in inflammation-associated cancer [83]. Furthermore, experimentations performed over two decades revealed that when human bronchial epithelial cells are exposed to high levels of nitric oxide (representative sources of RNS) which introduced superoxide ions, this resulted in transition mutations of the C:G pair to a T:A pair at the 248th codon of the *p53* gene [84]. Whereas, it can be observed that the chronic inflammation is leading the pathway towards carcinogenesis (Figure 2). It has been stated earlier in multiple literatures that at every stage of carcinogenesis, like cell multiplications, inhibition of senescence, resistance against anti-growth signals, and metastasis, chronic inflammation is the promoter for cancer [78,81]. Along with being mentioned as a promoter of cancer, it has also been made evident that in cells with chronic inflammation, there is a depravity of cell repair and cell death mechanisms, and instead of a promotion of abnormal cell proliferation [85].

Several immunomodulatory protein families are also implicated in inflammation. One such protein family is Siglecs [86]. Siglecs are receptors that are expressed on the surface of white blood cells and bind to sialic acids (Sia), a nine carbon atom monosaccharide [86–88]. Most members of this family carry an inhibitory motif and lead to the suppression of immune response [86–88]. Siglecs have been implicated in immunological response in many physiological and pathological conditions, including cancer [89–94]. In the case of a tumor, the cancer cells start to overexpress sialic acid, and the engagement of Siglecs on immune cells leads to immunoevasion and ultimately enhanced tumor growth [90,91]. A few members of the Siglec family are also activating in nature, and the engagement of these receptors leads to enhanced immune response and reduced tumor growth [92,95]. As priorly mentioned, oxidative stresses contributed by the inflammatory mediators and their by-products, seem to act as crucial protagonists in the development of carcinogenesis. Once inflammation-mediated cancer is established, it gears in pathways to strive onwards with the tumorigenic activities. One such pathway is the nuclear factor erythroid 2–related factor 2 (Nrf2) pathway that regulates the cancerous development.

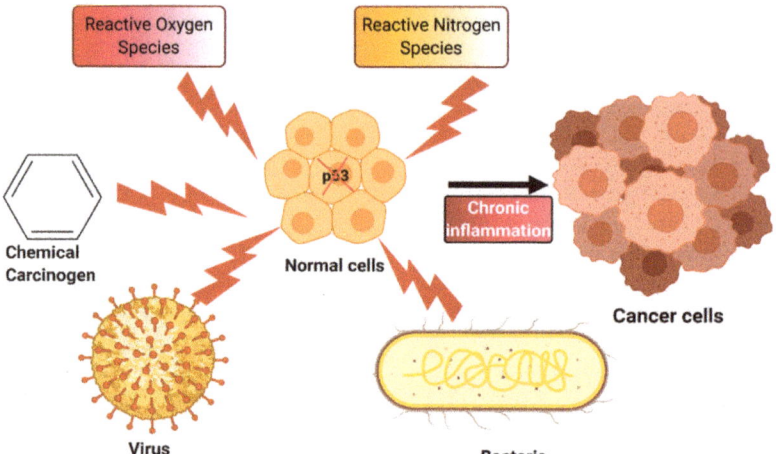

Figure 2. Chronic inflammation-induced carcinogenesis: The process of carcinogenesis sometimes involves chronic inflammation induced by chemical carcinogens, reactive oxygen and nitrogen species, viruses, and bacteria. All these agents trigger mutation in the *p53* gene that ultimately leads to the transformation of normal cells into cancer cells.

NRF2 Pathway and Its Role in Cancer

At normal conditions, Nrf2 acts as the transcription factor that binds the anti-oxidant response element (ARE) that initiates the expression of anti-oxidant and cytoprotective enzymes. The Nrf2 factor is maintained at a dormant phase by its negative regulator: the kelch-like ECH associated protein (Keap1)-Cullin 3 based ligase (CUL3) complex [96]. The Keap1-CUL3 complex sustains lower levels of Nrf2 by ubiquitination and proteasomal degradation, keeping it in a silenced phase [97]. Normally, Nrf2 is induced with increased oxidative stress, where it detaches from the Keap1-CUL3 complex, halting their antagonistic activity, enters the nucleus, binds to the ARE, and consequently expresses greater than 200 genes for anti-oxidative pathways [98]. However, in chronic inflammation-induced oxidative stress, the Nrf2 can escape its negative regulation performed by Keap1 by direct cause of increased oxidative stress that results in the upregulation of the p6 protein: an activator of Nrf2, and subsequently dismantles autophagocytosis of the p6 protein [99]. Nrf2 activity has been known to be exemplified by inhibiting the activities of Keap1 directly, such as p21Cip/WAF1, a competitive inhibitor of Keap1, inhibiting it from attaching to the DLG functional domain of Nrf2, thereby disrupting its ability of Nrf2 degradation [100]. Thus, it can be concluded that in chronic oxidative stresses, there is a hyper-regulation of Nrf2 activation. Similarly, when dealing with chronic inflammation-mediated cancers, there has been evidence that the Nrf2 factors are overexpressed, which could be due to mutations, changes in DNA methylation patterns, and protein alterations [101]. Carcinogenic promoting properties are harnessed by the Nrf2 in cancer cells, playing vicious roles in promoting cell proliferation, inhibiting apoptosis, and strengthening its resistance to chemo/radiotherapy [102]. One other interesting property imparted by Nrf2 to cancerous cells is drug resistance. It has been found in doxorubicin-resistant human ovarian cancer cells, the upregulation of Nrf2 resonates with its character of resistance [103]. Moreover, it has been described as a promoter of all the necessary key hallmarks needed to establish cancer, from increasing protein synthesis and expression of cell division genes to stimulating mRNA translations in support of cell proliferation [96].

5. Oxidative Stress, p53, and Inflammation

Oxidative stress is referred to as a state of imbalanced equilibrium between the generation of ROS with the anti-oxidant system of the body [104]. A balanced redox mechanism is necessary for maintaining genomic integrity. Excessive oxidative stress can cause immune dysfunction and, thereby, induce an inflammatory response. For instance, the immune cells, such as T lymphocyte activation, were found to be suppressed by excessive ROS leading to inflammation and tumorous conditions. ROS, therefore, plays a dual role by either suppressing T lymphocyte activation or its intermediate level modulate T lymphocyte differentiation at the site of injury. Contrastingly, a persistent level of ROS enhances apoptosis in T cell lymphocytes by damaging DNA through a p53 pathway [105]. Several methods have been adopted to sensitize T lymphocytes to the site of injury and inflammation. Amongst these, the use of polyphenol such as resveratrol was found to boost T lymphocytes significantly in mice by enhancing CD86 and MHC-II antigens [106]. Another phytochemical, lycopene, alleviates oxidative injury in ruminant animals by inhibiting inflammatory cytokines and apoptosis. The anti-oxidant potential of lycopene ameliorates hydrogen peroxide (H_2O_2)-induced inflammation by regulating the Nrf2-ARE pathway in primary bMEC and MAC-T cells [107].

Further, in vivo studies have also shown a correlation between increased oxidative stress leading to neurobehavioral disorders. Buthionine sulfoximine (BSO)-induced oxidative stress in BTBR T$^+$ tf/J (BTBR) mice have resulted in depletion of the native enzymatic anti-oxidant system, which has resulted in autism-like repetitive behaviors [108]. A systemic review also suggested that an imbalanced redox potential may contribute to neurodegenerative diseases by altering differentiation and the number of CD4$^+$ T cell subpopulations [109]. Several reports indicated that oxidative stress-mediated inflammation could lead to cancer progression. Activation of transcription factors including NF-κB, AP-1, p53, HIF-1α, PPAR-γ, β-catenin/Wnt, and Nrf2 can transform normal cells into cancerous cells. Furthermore, a cross-talk between NF-κB activation and cell proliferation regulates the immunological and inflammatory response resulting in tumor conditions [110]. Such reports also indicated the possibility of using NF-κB as a prognostic marker to identify cancers, in particular, colon cancer [111]. It is noteworthy to observe that these transcriptional factors mediate p53-dependent fashion in response to an inflammatory condition.

Oxidative stress-induced p53 activation is common in inflammation and cancers. Activation of p53 primarily regulates the cell cycle, DNA repair, and apoptotic mechanisms [112]. Cancer cells exhibit higher ROS levels than normal cells since they are serving as an oncogenic agent with increased metabolism and mutation rates [113]. DNA damage caused by chemotherapeutic drugs, environmental and chemical toxins, radiations, and immunosuppressive drugs often elevates ROS levels, leading to p53 activation. Homeostatic regulation of ROS and p53 is necessary to determine the fate of normal tissue stem cells. Recent data have shown the direct relationship between ROS and p53 for the differentiation of stem cells. The lack of p53 functioning in the neural progenitor cells leads to increased ROS and premature differentiation [114]. Meanwhile, restoring ectopic expression of p53, and with anti-oxidants, enhances partial differentiation and stemness [115]. Many data have shown the dual mode of p53 functioning depending on the nature, duration, and intensity of oxidative stress imposed in different cell types. Hence, either anti-oxidant or pro-oxidant regulatory functioning of p53 is well known, depending on the type of cell burden. Activation of p53 by anti-oxidants imposes a protective mechanism against oxidative stress by ameliorating excessive ROS levels in the cells. Further, both endogenous and exogenous supply of anti-oxidants could play a role in inhibiting adhesion and invasion properties of cancer cells [116,117]. In contrast, pro-oxidants exert oxidative stress-induced p53 functioning leading to autophagy, caspase-mediated apoptosis, and necrotic cell death mechanisms [118,119]. A detailed analysis of anti-oxidant versus pro-oxidant effects on p53 mediated functioning is discussed elsewhere [116,120].

6. Plant Flavonoids as Therapeutic Agents

Over the last two decades, plant polyphenols, especially flavonoids, have gained significant attention in developing treatments for disorders such as Parkinson's disease, inflammatory bowel disease, Alzheimer's disease, obesity, cancer, and cardiovascular diseases (CVDs) [121,122]. A plethora of research has been done already to show how flavonoids influence these diseased conditions, mostly with their biochemical and pharmacological properties such as pro-oxidant and anti-oxidant potentials that correlates to their structure–activity relationship. Plant flavonoids share a basic structure of diphenyl propane in which two benzene rings are connected through a pyran ring. The subclasses of flavonoids such as flavones, flavonols, isoflavones, anthocyanin, flavan-3-ols, and flavanones differ by the attachment of carbon on the C ring to which the B ring is attached (Figure 3) [123]. Further, the degree of unsaturation and oxidation of the C ring contributes to the different classifications of flavonoids.

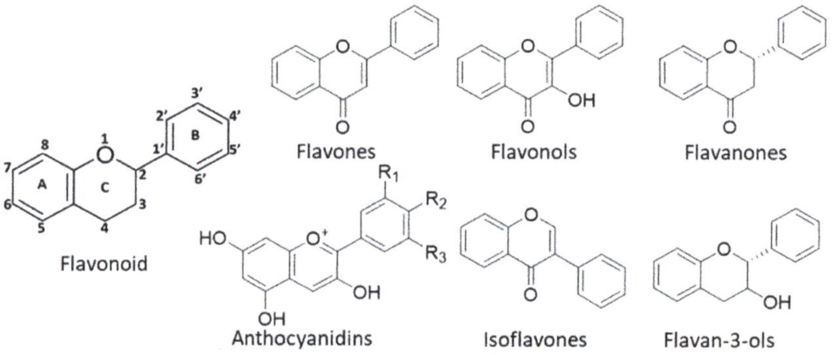

Figure 3. Basic structure of a flavonoid and its subclasses.

The structure-activity relationship of flavonoids majorly attributes to their observed clinical effects both in in vitro and in vivo studies. For instance, an anti-oxidant property of a flavonoid largely depends on the functional group it possesses and its spatial arrangement around the nucleus. The importance of the B ring and the hydroxyl group at position 3 often contributes to ROS scavenging potentials, as evident by the experimental and theoretical derivations. Furthermore, this spatial arrangement of the functional group and its substitution, along with the number of sugar moieties (glycosides) and hydroxyl groups, determines the mechanism of anti-oxidant potentials observed for several flavonoids [124,125]. Anti-oxidants exert various radical scavenging properties either by inhibiting chelated trace elements or enzymes that generate excessive ROS and/or by enhancing endogenous anti-oxidant enzymes such as glutathione peroxidase (GPx), catalase (CAT), and superoxide dismutase (SOD). In contrast, the pro-oxidant effect of flavonoids can result in preventing cancer through inhibiting the proliferation of tumor cells with apoptotic induction. Recent structure–activity studies have shown that the flavonoids possess significant anti-proliferative effects, especially in the presence of di-OH 3', 4', a double bond at C2-C3 and a carbonyl at the C4 position. However, flavonoids that possess functional chemical moiety at the C7-C8 position showed low to non-significant anti-proliferative effects [126]. These observations further warrant discussions on the importance of flavonoids in treating disease, especially inflammation and cancer, which are discussed below.

7. Flavonoids in Inflammation and Cancer Prevention

The p53-mediated pathway has been an attractive target for many of the flavonoids in regulating inflammation and cancers. Flavonoids regulate transcription factors such as NF-κB, Nrf2, and AP-1 in inflammation and DNA damage, cell cycle, and apoptosis in tumor cell proliferation. We have reviewed dietary flavonoids such as quercetin, luteolin, cyanidin, daidzein, and epigallocatechin gallate (EGCG) along with other flavonoids, which showed promising results in preclinical and clinical trials. While many reviews are available on discussing how different flavonoids can be used to induce apoptosis in cancer models, we have focused on flavonoids and their ability to prevent inflammation and cancers with a focus on p53-mediated mechanisms.

7.1. Quercetin

Quercetin, a flavonol found in vegetables and fruits, has been reported for various pharmacological properties that include scavenging ROS, inhibiting inflammation, and preventing cancer. One of the mechanisms by which quercetin exerts cytoprotective effects is through regulating MEK/ERK and Keap1/Nrf2/ARE pathways in inflammation [127]. An in vitro study has shown the protective effect of quercetin in cigarette smoke extract-induced inflammation by downregulating cytokine markers such as IL-1β, IL-6, and IL-8 in ARPE-19 cells. Pretreatment with quercetin further activates the Keap1/Nrf2/ARE-anti-oxidant pathway, which induces cellular defenses against various oxidative stress [128]. Recent reports have shown that p53 can activate the Keap1/Nrf2/ARE-anti-oxidant pathway and can act as the main regulator of the cells anti-oxidant response [129,130]. This effect of p53 largely depends on the intensity and degree of oxidative stress imposed. A lower level of oxidative stress has been correlated with increased anti-oxidant enzymes, such as SOD and CAT [131]. A flavonoid-rich extract from *Rosa laevigata* Michx fruit exerts neuroprotective effects by downregulating the levels of p-JNK, p-ERK, and p-p38 in MAPK pathways [132]. Furthermore, various in vivo studies in mice and rats have shown the downregulation of anti-inflammatory markers with increased anti-oxidant defense proteins (SOD, CAT, GPx) under oxidative stress-induced conditions, such as adipose hypertrophy, hepatocarcinogenesis, and obesity-induced skeletal muscle inflammation [133,134]. Further, quercetin significantly reduces adipocyte size and enhanced angiogenesis and adipogenesis by downregulating TNFα and HIF-1 α levels along with proteins such as TLR-4, CD68, MCP-1, and JNK [135].

Quercetin has been extensively studied to explore its mechanism of action in cancer prevention. Treatment with quercetin was reported to protect DNA damage induced by H_2O_2 in human Caco-2 cells. Quercetin decreases single-strand DNA breaks by enhancing the expression of human 8-oxoguanine DNA glycosylase and DNA repair mechanisms [136]. However, the detailed mechanism of p53 involvement in cancer prevention by quercetin remains unclear. It is believed that upon regulating p53 mechanisms, quercetin possesses a dual role and can have better control over cellular events to mitigate oxidative stress imposed by carcinogens through activating the Keap1/Nrf2/ARE anti-oxidant pathway and/or inducing apoptosis. In a recent study by Wang et al., quercetin was able to inhibit apoptosis by downregulating p53, Bax, and caspase-3 expression in ARPE-19 cells, and, thereby, it prevents high glucose-induced injury [137]. A similar kind of protective effect was also noted in the study by Darband et al., in which quercetin was able to inhibit oxidative DNA damage by activating the Nrf2 signaling pathway. Supplementation of quercetin (50 mg/kg) in rats reduces colon carcinogenesis induced by 1,2-dimethylhydrazine (DMH) [138]. In contrast, a study by Clemente-Soto et al., demonstrated the activation of p53 upon quercetin treatment in cervical cancer cells leading to apoptosis and DNA damage [139]. There are several reports available to demonstrate the similar functioning of p53-induced apoptosis, leading to cancer growth inhibition and prevention. This could be attributed to the multiple facts that the quercetin binding potentials to several receptors that may be important in the prevention of carcinogenesis, induces epigenetic modifiers, and interferes with enzymes such as native anti-oxidants, to elicit its protective mechanisms. Despite these properties, quercetin could sensitize and protect noncancerous cells during chemotherapy or radiotherapy when used in combination with existing classes of cancer chemotherapeutic-drugs [140].

7.2. Luteolin

Luteolin, a flavone found in many plants such as *Salvia tomentosa* Mill. (Balsamic sage) and *Glossogyne tenuifolia* possess anti-inflammatory effects via downregulating the NF-κB pathway. Luteolin was found to inhibit inflammation induced by infectious pathogens such as *Staphylococcus aureus* to cause mastitis. Treatment with luteolin reduces cytokines expression such as TNF-α, IL-1β, and IL-6 in a mouse model mimicking mastitis. Furthermore, luteolin suppressed the expression of IκBα and NF-κB, along with matrix metalloprotease-2 (MMP-2) and MMP-9, to render protection against inflammation [141]. A recent report showed the protective effect of luteolin against testicular deficits caused by lead acetate. Luteolin (50 mg/kg) treatment in male Wistar rats significantly activates the Nrf2/HO-1 pathway by increasing native anti-oxidant enzymes and inhibits inflammatory and apoptotic cascades [142]. These protective effects could relate to the anti-oxidant potential of luteolin [143] and it's functioning on the p53 protein, as it is suppressed in *Staphylococcus aureus*-induced inflammation, preventing apoptosis [144]. Furthermore, a study by Li et al., proved the anti-oxidant nature of luteolin by activating the Nrf2 signaling pathway and NF-κB-mediated inflammatory responses in type 1 diabetes in mice. Modulation of these pathways reduces MMP protein expression and cellular hypertrophy [145]. These studies show that the protective effect of luteolin against inflammation largely depends on its anti-oxidant nature rather than its pro-oxidant effect, which inhibits different cancer cell proliferation [143].

Luteolin exerts its cancer-preventive properties by inhibiting DNA damage and activating anti-oxidant mechanisms in a p53 regulated manner. Combinational treatment of luteolin and EGCG showed translocation of p53 to the mitochondria, thereby regulating apoptosis [146]. This translocation of p53 is crucial and depends on the degree of stress burden imposed. The mitochondrial translocation occurs if the damage or stress is irreversible [147]. Further, in a study by Jiang et al., luteolin exerts its tumor-preventive potential by regulating the expression of microRNAs (miRNAs). Treatment in non-small cell lung cancer cell lines reduced cell proliferation and tumor inhibition in the H460 xenograft tumor model. The expression of an enhanced miR-34a-5p level was observed in tumor tissues, which resulted in a reduced level of MDM4 proteins. Furthermore, luteolin treatment enhanced p53 and p21 expression and reduced tumorigenesis [148]. The isolated compound luteolin from *Melissa officinalis* L, showed DNA damage protective effects induced by ultraviolet B radiation (UVB) in skin cells. Treatment with luteolin reduced DNA double strand breaks and the DNA damage response (DDR) mechanism in these cells [149]. Many studies have shown the upregulation of p53-mediated apoptosis for tumor inhibition in various cancer cell lines [150,151] and are not in the scope for this review.

7.3. EGCG

An anti-oxidant potent flavan-3-ol, EGCG, mostly seen in green tea polyphenols, showed anti-inflammatory effects under imposed oxidative stress conditions. EGCG exhibited an anti-inflammatory effect by inhibiting pro-inflammatory cytokines', p53, NF-κB, TLRs, and STAT3 expression. In a recent study by Wang et al., rats were administrated with EGCG (50 mg/kg) and analyzed for parameters for anxiety-like behavior and myocardial infarction. ELISA and PCR studies have shown a significant reduction of IL-6 along with STAT3 expression. Further, inhibition of apoptosis cascades (caspase expression) was observed in rats. Hence, the intake of EGCG reversed anxiety-like behavior and prevented inflammation [152]. Similar observations were made by Ren et al., wherein lipopolysaccharides (LPS)-induced retinal inflammation in rats was attenuated by green tea extract (containing EGCG) through inhibiting phosphorylation of STAT3 and NF-κB along with pro-inflammatory cytokines [153]. Further reports have shown a strong association between EGCG and TLRs, which play an important role in the host immune system. TLR4 has a strong relation with inflammatory response and cancer progression [154]. It is interesting to observe that the p53-mediated differential expression of TLR4 depends on the context of the cells. In p53 wild type cells, the activation of TLR4 results in type-I IFN (IFN-γ) secretion, resulting in p21 mediated cell cycle arrest. Whereas in p53 mutant cells, the activation of TLR4 promotes cancer [58]. EGCG was shown to inhibit TLR4 expression in in vitro and in vivo studies [155,156]. However, EGCG's direct involvement in p53-mediated regulation of TLR4 is not fully understood.

EGCG, being an active anti-oxidant, protects DNA damage mediated cell death in many cells. As observed for other flavonoids, EGCG exerts its preventive potentials by modulating Nrf2 and JAK/STAT pathways in testicular ischemia reperfusion injury-induced oxidative damage. Pre-perfusion treatment with EGCG prevented phosphorylation of JAK2, STAT3, and STAT1 along with apoptotic markers [157]. Likewise, EGCG prevents apoptosis and astrogliosis induced by acrylamide in rats. Pretreatment in rats with EGCG showed reduced DNA fragmentation, Bax, Bcl-2, caspase 3, and cytochrome c expression. Further, EGCG enhanced native anti-oxidant enzymes and glutathione levels to mitigate excessive ROS production [158]. EGCG was also shown to modulate DNA methylation processes, especially DNA methyltransferase 1, thereby rendering DNA protection [159]. Genomic stability of the cells can be safeguarded against various carcinogens by consuming flavonoids. Detailed mechanisms on DNA damage response and prevention are discussed elsewhere [160,161].

7.4. Cyanidin

Cyanidin, an anthocyanidin, found in plant pigments and berries [162] including grapes, bilberry, and blackberry, has been found to possess anti-inflammatory effects under oxidative stress conditions. Cyanidin-3-glucoside (C3G) is a naturally occurring anthocyanin in plants and cyanidin is the aglycone of C3G. Both C3G and cyanidin have shown significant anti-inflammatory effects against 2, 4, 6-trinitrobenzenesulfonic acid (TNBS)-induced colitis in mice. Administration of 200 μmol/kg in mice reduces inflammatory markers (TNF-α, IL-1β, IL-6, and interferon-γ) and thereby protecting the intestinal barrier [163]. Similarly, in vitro effects have been studied on Caco-2 cells, which showed inhibition in the disruption of intestinal barrier dysfunction. Further, C3G was found to improve diabetic conditions, especially diabetic nephropathy (DN). Eight weeks supplementation of 10–20 mg/kg of C3G in rats improves native oxidative enzymes and modulate the TGF-β1/Smad2/3 pathway to render renal protection [164]. This effect was further improved by encapsulating C3G in chitosan nanoparticles for targeted drug delivery and resulted in p53 mediated protection in mice. C3G downregulated p53-mediated apoptosis in mice with a balanced B-cell lymphoma-2/leukemia-2 ratio [165].

Further, C3G rendered DNA damage protection in BEAS-2B and HaCaT cells in vitro from oxidative stress imposed by nitrosamine, 4-(methylnitrosamino)-1-(3-pyridyl)-1-butanone (NNK) and UVB, respectively. In both studies, the degree of DNA damage was decreased by modulating ATM/ATR pathways, which is mediated by p53 expression [166,167]. Treatment with C3G restores the Bcl-2 expression in HaCaT cells and inhibits caspase-3 activation. Our previous study on apple peel flavonoid fraction (AF4) containing C3G as the main constituent, showed a DNA protective effect on NNK, methotrexate (MTX), and cisplatin-induced toxicity in BEAS-2B cells. Pretreatment with AF4 reduced the ROS level with an increase in anti-oxidant enzymes. Further, AF4 reduces DNA damage and enhanced protection against carcinogens by facilitating DNA repair mechanisms [168]. A study by Kaewmool et al., showed both anti-inflammatory and apoptotic effects of C3G in PC-12 cells. Anti-inflammation was mediated by decreased expression of IL-1β and IL-6 along with inducible nitric oxide synthase (iNOS) and Cox2 expression, while the apoptotic effect was mediated by a caspase-3 induced mechanism [169].

7.5. Daidzein

Daidzein, an isoflavone, found in soybeans and soy products, is known to possess anti-inflammatory and cancer-preventive properties by inhibiting various inflammatory cytokines and cell death markers, respectively. Daidzein was found to inhibit the nephrotoxicity posed by cisplatin-induced oxidative stress in proximal tubular cells of mice. Treatment with daidzein inhibits the expression of TNFα, IL-10, and IL-18 along with enhanced anti-oxidant defense enzymes (SOD and GPx) activity. Further, daidzein reduces kidney injury markers (NGAL, BUN, creatinine, and KIM-1) and cell death mechanisms (caspase-3/7) [170]. Daidzein also improves the adverse effect of adipose inflammation by regulating the proliferator-activated receptor γ (PPARγ) in 3T3-L1 adipocytes. A decreased expression of monocyte chemoattractant protein-1 (MCP-1) and TNF-α was noted in adipose tissue of daidzein-fed mice [171]. Similar effects were observed by Feng et al., wherein daidzein treatment in rats inhibited TLR4 and NF-κB activation leading to the prevention of inflammation [172]. Furthermore, the synergic effect of daidzein and genistein exerts photoprotective potentials by regulating growth arrest and DNA damage (gadd45) genes, to decrease DNA damage and enhances DNA repair process in UV-induced photodamage [173,174]. The possible mechanisms by which flavonoids exert their anti-inflammatory and cancer-preventive properties are illustrated in Figure 4. Other flavonoids and their anti-inflammatory and cancer-prevention properties are summarized in Table 1.

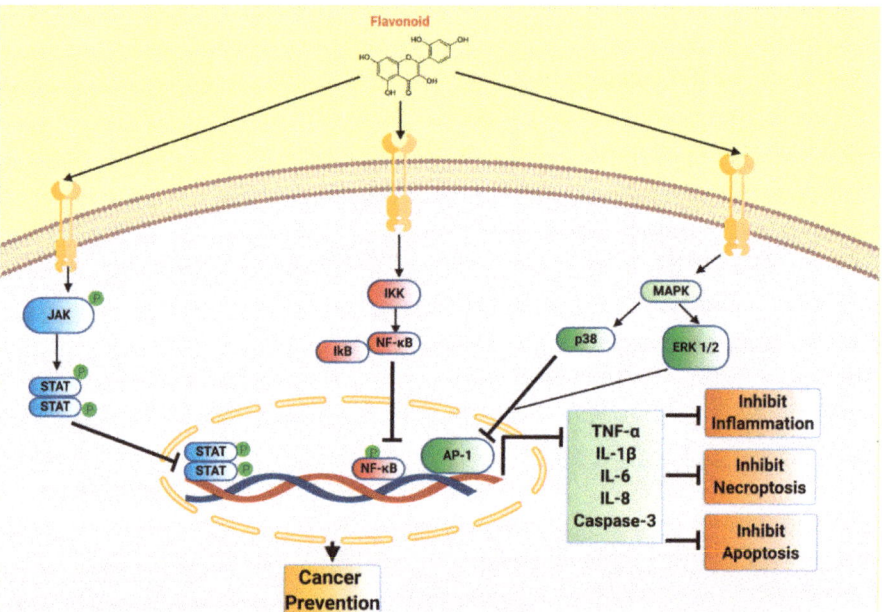

Figure 4. Flavonoids inhibiting inflammatory and cancer markers: The flavonoids can modulate several receptors and their corresponding signaling cascades. The flavonoids exert its effects mainly through JAK/STAT, IKK/NF-κB, and MAPK pathways leading to inhibition of pro-inflammatory, pro-apoptotic, and pro-necroptosis markers. The effector molecules that are downregulated include cytokines and cell death markers such as IL-1β, TNF-α, IL-6, IL-8, caspase-3, etc. These cellular events ultimately lead to immune regulation and cancer prevention.

Table 1. Flavonoids in preventing inflammation and cancer in preclinical and experimental cell models.

Flavonoid	Disease/Oxidative Stress Imposed	Preclinical or Cell Model	Molecular Signaling/Pathway	Inflammation/Cancer Prevention Status	Reference
Apigenin	Cardiotoxicity	Rats	Decreases caspase-3 and Bax	Inhibition of apoptosis	[175]
	Myocardial injury	Mice	Inhibits TNF-α, IL-1β, MIP-1α, MIP-2, and NFκB	Inhibit inflammation	[176]
	UVB-induced skin cancer	Mice	Inhibits IL-6 and IL-12	Inhibit inflammation	[177]
	Bowel disease and colitis-associated cancer	Mice and HCT-116	Inhibits STAT3 and NF-κB	Inhibit inflammation-induced carcinogenesis	[178]
	Isoproterenol hydrochloride-induced apoptosis	H9C2	Inhibits Bax, caspase-3, -8, and -9 and cytochrome c	Cancer prevention	[179]
Chrysin	Cerebral ischemia	Rats	Inhibits IL-1β and TNF-α	Inhibit inflammation	[180]
	Cerebral ischemia	Rats	Inhibits TNF-α, IL-6, and IL-1β; activates PI3K/Akt/mTOR pathway	Inhibit inflammation and apoptosis	[181]
	Reproductive toxicity	Mice	Inhibits IL-1β, TNF-α, IL-6, and IL-10; activates caspase 3 and 9	Inhibit inflammation	[182]
	Hepatic encephalopathy	Rats	Increases glutathione level; inhibit NF-κB, TNF-α, IL-6, and TLR-4; reduces caspase-3 and hepatic necrosis	Inhibit inflammation and apoptosis	[183]
Daidzein	Endometriosis	OESCs and NESCs	Inhibited IL-6, IL-8, COX-2, TNF-α-induced IκB phosphorylation and p65	Inhibit inflammation	[184]
	Intestinal mucositis	Mice	Inhibits TNF-α, IL-1β, and IL-6; increases CAT and GPx level	Inhibit inflammation	[185]
Naringenin	Obesity	Mice	Inhibits TLRs and TNF-α	Inhibit inflammation	[186]
	Pulmonary metastasis	Mice	Inhibits Tgf-β1	Cancer prevention	[187]
	Cardiac hypercholesterolemia	Rats	Inhibits DNA damage, TNF-α, and RIP3	Inhibits necroptosis	[188]

Table 1. Cont.

Flavonoid	Disease/Oxidative Stress Imposed	Preclinical or Cell Model	Molecular Signaling/Pathway	Inflammation/Cancer Prevention Status	Reference
Kaempferol	Propacetamol-induced acute liver injury	Mice	Inhibits cytochrome P450 2E1; restores SOD, GPx and CAT; inhibits Bax/Bcl-2 ratio	Prevents apoptosis	[189]
	Etoposide-induced oxidative stress	HL-60 and PBMCs	Inhibits DNA damage (tail length)	Prevents DNA damage	[190]
	Paw Edema	Mice and THP-1 (together)	Inhibits Cox-2; STAT3 and NF-κB	Inhibit inflammation	[191]
	Brain Injury and neuroinflammation	Rats	Inhibits STAT3 and NF-κB p65	Inhibit inflammation	[189]
Fisetin	Hypoxia	NCI-H157	Inhibit HIF 1-α and STAT3	Prevents hypoxia	[192]
	Hydrogen peroxide-induced oxidative stress	HaCaT	Inhibits iNOS, Cox-2, IL-1β, IL-6, and TNF-α	Inhibit inflammation	[193]
	Diabetic cardiomyopathy	Rats	Restores SOD and CAT; inhibits IL-1β, IL-6, and TNF-α; inhibits caspase-3, Bax, and Bax/Bcl-2 ratio	Inhibit inflammation and apoptosis	[194]
Myricetin	LPS-induced Inflammation	Mice and RAW 264.7	Inhibits NF-κB p65 and AKT activation	Inhibit inflammation	[195]
	Colonic chronic-induced inflammation	Mice	Inhibits TNF-α, IL-1β, IL-6, NF-κB, p-NF-κB, cyclooxygenase-2 (COX-2), PCNA, and Cyclin D1	Inhibits inflammation and tumor	[196]
Hesperetin	Hepatic fibrosis	Mice and HSCs	Inhibit α-SMA, Col1α1, Col3α1 and TIMP-1	Inhibits inflammation and induce apoptosis	[197]
	Testicular Damage	Rats	Inhibits malondialdehyde, ROS, DNA fragmentation, and caspase 3; inhibits TNFα and IL-17	Inhibits inflammation and apoptosis	[198]
Catechin	TNF-α-induced inflammation	3T3-L1	Inhibit IL-1α, IL-1β, IL-6, IL-12, p35, iNOS, Cox-2, NF-κB, AMPK, FOXO3a, and SIRT1	Inhibits inflammation	[199]
	Methylglyoxal-induced cytotoxicity	EA.hy926	Inhibits MMP and cytotoxicity	Inhibits apoptosis	[200]

8. Flavonoids and Dietary Intake

Recent epidemiological, cross-sectional and short-term randomized controlled studies have proved a direct relationship between flavonoid-rich diet intake and health benefits resulting in preventing various diseases. Flavonoids, with numerous potentials, as discussed above, improve life-threatening conditions, particularly cancer and CVDs. This direct correlation is based on several factors such as type/composition of flavonoid(s), their bioavailability after consumption, and the epidemiological region.

For instance, the average intake of flavan-3-ol among Europeans ranges between 77 mg/day to 182 mg/day probably because of the high consumption of tea, at least in the UK [201]. A large portion of ingested flavan-3-ol remained in the large intestine as they are not readily absorbed by phase II conjugating enzymes. This availability of flavan-3-ol could benefit microbiota in the colon region to metabolize further into monomers and contribute to an enhanced immune system [202,203]. In other countries of Europe (except the UK), a rich flavan-3-ol diet was mostly observed because of the consumption of non-citrus fruits (apples/pears) [201]. A meta-analysis of epidemiologic studies has shown a positive correlation between the consumption of flavan-3-ol and reduced cancer. The higher consumption of flavan-3-ol reduces rectal, oropharyngeal, breast, and laryngeal cancers [204]. In contrast, a study among 38,408 women aged ≥45 y with a frequent diet enriched with flavonols did not correlate with cancer risk prevention. The best explanation for the discrepancy could be due to a relatively low range of flavonoid intake combined with populations free of CVDs and cancers. However, continuous efforts have been made to overcome such issues as well as lipophilic nature, low solubility, and variable bioavailability of flavonoids by introducing different formulations to nanocrystals technology [205].

Another intake of flavonoids, such as anthocyanins and flavanones, exhibited a lower risk of CVDs in both women and men. A study conducted in 43,880 healthy men who have the habit of consuming a higher anthocyanin intake showed a lower risk of developing ischemic stroke over a period of 24 y [206]. Various studies have shown that the anthocyanins exert healthy beneficial effects on LDL-cholesterol level, which is mediated by cholesterol efflux capacity [207]. In a randomized controlled trial, anthocyanins showed anti-inflammatory effects by reducing hypercholesterolemic conditions in adults. This effect was consistent with previous observations as intake of anthocyanins significantly reduced LDL-cholesterol and HDL-cholesterol levels with inhibition of IL-6 and IL-1β in a HepG2 cell line [208]. It is noteworthy to observe that a mixture of anthocyanins was more effective than individual components for improved human health. As discussed earlier, it could be the anti-oxidant potential of flavonoids that might exert these effects, as observed from a recent cross-sectional study conducted in the Italian population against the human papillomavirus (hrHPV) infection. The study was conducted in 251 women with normal cervical cytology, showed a significant reduction in the risk of developing hrHPV infection with anthocyanins-rich diet [209]. Further, a flavonoid-rich diet has been studied for their protective effects against various disease conditions which are shown in Table 2.

Moreover, the dietary intake of flavonoids has a direct impact with microbiota as ingested flavonoids are known to be unabsorbed in the proximal intestine, further reach the colon region. This microenvironment facilitates the hydrolysis and fermentation of flavonoids employing different enzymes released by the microorganisms. Microbes can facilitate oxidation, demethylation, and catabolism of flavonoids into phenolic acids and aromatic catabolites [210]. Recent studies have shown that the high flavonoid-rich diet exerts an inverse correlation with obesity and inflammation. This is largely mediated by gut microbiota as it increases adiposity and fatty acid metabolism. Further, intestinal microbes modify flavonoids by glucosidation, dihydroxylation, and decarboxylation converting them into monomers, which can be more absorbable in the intestine [211]. To add, flavonoids isolated from mulberry leaves ameliorate lipid dysmetabolism in the high fat diet (HFD)-fed mice. Gut microbes such as *Bacteroidetes* played a role in the increased production of acetic acid, thereby restoring lipid metabolism [212]. From these observations, it is noteworthy to believe that both classifications of flavonoids and microbiota play a cross-talk between dietary intake and improved health benefits.

Table 2. Flavonoids-rich diet in disease prevention: a summary from recent (2019–2020) clinical trials.

Dietary Flavonoids	Condition Studied	Sample Details	Key Observations	Reference
Seidlitzia Rosmarinus (flavonoid-rich)	Recurrent cystitis	126 women	Lowered symptoms of cystitis; prevent the incidence of recurrent cystitis with no side effects	[213]
Genistein with FOLFOX	Metastatic colorectal cancer	13 patients	Exposure of genistein with FOLFOX was safe and tolerable	[214]
Anthocyanin-rich blueberry	Type 2 diabetes and CVD	115 people	Improved endothelial function, systemic arterial stiffness and attenuated cyclic guanosine monophosphate concentrations	[215]
Anthocyanin-rich fruit juice	Healthy volunteers	57 males	Demonstrated DNA-protective and anti-oxidant effects; reduction in body fat and an increase in fat-free mass with increased SOD level	[216]
Flavonoid-rich natural cocoa beverage	Plasma oxidative stress and inflammation	134 people	Improved glycemia, triglyceridemia, high-density lipoprotein cholesterol, low-density lipoprotein cholesterol, triglyceridemia/HDL index, and oxidative markers	[217]
Genistein	Human prostate cancer	14 males	Increased Brain Abundant Membrane Attached Signal Protein 1(BASP1) expression; decreases MMP-2 in prostate tissue	[218]
EGCG	Acute radiation-induced esophagitis (ARIE)	83 patients	Lowered ARIE by reducing acute pain index (API) and acute dysphagia index (ADI) without side effects	[219]
EGCG	Cutaneous scarring	62 humans	Reduced mast cells; down-regulated Vascular Endothelial Growth Factor A (VEGFA) and CD31; reduced scar thickness	[220]
Quercetin	Eccentric exercise-induced muscle damage	12 males	Increased the isometric strength for contraction; lower torque and muscle fiber conduction velocity; attenuate the severity of muscle weakness	[221]
Silymarin	Radiation-induced dermatitis	40 patients	Delayed in radiodermatitis development and progression	[222]

9. Conclusions and Future Directions

The role of p53 in inflammation and cancer is well established. Being a central protein in immune pathways, the modulation of p53 expression may lead to the prevention of many diseases. Further cross-talk between p53 and immune checkpoints, such as MHC1 and TLRs, has great potential in developing drugs, especially for cancer immunotherapy. As discussed in this review, flavonoids are one of the ideal choices of biomolecules for developing safer immunosuppresses in the management of chronic inflammation leading to cancer progression. Many of the flavonoids exert their preventive potentials by enhancing the endogenous anti-oxidant system through modulating the Keap1/Nrf2/ARE pathway. Although the p53-mediated Nrf2 pathway is not well studied, there is evidence to show that the activation of the Nrf2 pathway leads to a reduction in oxidative stress and enhanced DNA repair processes [223]. Thus flavonoids, especially with anti-oxidant properties, enhance the immune response against various oxidative stress-mediated cellular malfunctions leading to disease prevention. Further, a flavonoid-rich diet has shown evidence for the above cytoprotective mechanism in recent clinical trials, showing their disease-preventive potential.

However, direct links between flavonoid-mediated p53 and the anti-oxidant Keap1/Nrf2/ARE pathway to exert preventive potentials are scarce. In contrast, many reports have shown a p53-mediated induction of cell death pathways that can be regulated by flavonoids in various cancer models. Further, exploring the role of flavonoids through the p53 pathway in disease prevention should be of great interest for future research. Understanding the safe and efficacious dose of flavonoids is also very crucial in treatment since most flavonoids, depending on the concentration and microenvironment, can act as either anti-oxidants or prooxidants exhibiting hormetic effects. Moreover, continuous efforts are in progress for enhancing the bioavailability of flavonoids by acylation to enhance cellular uptake, improving stability by using different formulations, engineering microbiota for their improved impacts, and developing technologies, such as nanocrystals, for enhanced pharmacokinetics and targeted therapy.

Funding: This work received no external funding.

Acknowledgments: The authors thank the American University of Ras Al Khaimah (AURAK) for providing the infrastructure and facilities for the successful accomplishment of this project. Figure 1, Figure 2, and Figure 3 were created with BioRender.com. The authors would like to thank Andrea Verhagen, Cellular and Molecular Medicine, University of California, San Diego, USA, for proofreading the article.

Conflicts of Interest: The authors declare no conflict of interest.

Abbreviations

AID	activation-induced cytidine deaminase
AOM	azoxymethane
AP1	activator protein 1
ARE	anti-oxidant response element
ATP	adenosine triphosphate
BSO	buthionine sulfoximine
Cag-A	cytotoxin-associated gene A
Cat	catalase
CIA	collagen-induced arthritis
CNS	central nervous system
CVD	cardiovascular diseases
DDR	DNA damage response
DMH	1,2-dimethylhydrazine
EAE	experimental autoimmune encephalomyelitis
EGCG	epigallocatechin gallate
ERAP	endoplasmic reticulum aminopeptidase 1
HCC	hepatocellular carcinoma
HFD	high fat diet
HIF1	hypoxia inducible factor
IKK	IκB kinase
IPM	immune prognostic model
LFS	Li-Fraumeni syndrome
LOH	loss of heterozygosity
LPS	lipopolysaccharides
M-CSF	macrophage colony-stimulating factor
MHC	major histocompatibility complex
MMP	matrix metalloprotease

NF-κB	nuclear factor-κB
NRF2	nuclear factor erythroid 2-related factor 2
PAMPs	pathogen-associated molecular patterns
PPAR	peroxisome proliferator-activated receptors
PTEN	phosphatase and tensin homolog
ROS	Reactive oxygen species
SOCS1	suppressors of cytokine signaling 1
SOD	superoxide dismutase
STAT3	signal transducer and activator of transcription 3
TAM	tumor-associated macrophage
TAP1	transporter associated with Antigen Processing 1
TLR	toll-like receptor
TNBS	2,4,6-trinitrobenzenesulfonic acid
UVB	ultraviolet B radiation
WT	wild type

References

1. Hanahan, D.; Weinberg, R.A. Hallmarks of cancer: The next generation. *Cell* **2011**, *144*, 646–674. [CrossRef] [PubMed]
2. Jackson, S.P.; Bartek, J. The DNA-damage response in human biology and disease. *Nature* **2009**, *461*, 1071–1078. [CrossRef] [PubMed]
3. Freed-Pastor, W.A.; Prives, C. Mutant p53: One name, many proteins. *Genes Dev.* **2012**, *26*, 1268–1286. [CrossRef] [PubMed]
4. Levine, A.J.; Oren, M. The first 30 years of p53: Growing ever more complex. *Nat. Rev. Cancer* **2009**, *9*, 749–758. [CrossRef] [PubMed]
5. Lane, D.P. Cancer. p53, guardian of the genome. *Nature* **1992**, *358*, 15–16. [CrossRef]
6. Ben David, Y.; Prideaux, V.R.; Chow, V.; Benchimol, S.; Bernstein, A. Inactivation of the p53 oncogene by internal deletion or retroviral integration in erythroleukemic cell lines induced by Friend leukemia virus. *Oncogene* **1988**, *3*, 179–185.
7. Wolf, D.; Rotter, V. Inactivation of p53 gene expression by an insertion of Moloney murine leukemia virus-like DNA sequences. *Mol. Cell. Biol.* **1984**, *4*, 1402–1410. [CrossRef]
8. Baker, S.J.; Fearon, E.R.; Nigro, J.M.; Hamilton, S.R.; Preisinger, A.C.; Jessup, J.M.; Van Tuinen, P.; Ledbetter, D.H.; Barker, D.F.; Nakamura, Y.; et al. Chromosome 17 deletions and p53 gene mutations in colorectal carcinomas. *Science* **1989**, *244*, 217–221. [CrossRef]
9. Petitjean, A.; Mathe, E.; Kato, S.; Ishioka, C.; Tavtigian, S.V.; Hainaut, P.; Olivier, M. Impact of mutant p53 functional properties on TP53 mutation patterns and tumor phenotype: Lessons from recent developments in the IARC TP53 database. *Hum. Mutat.* **2007**, *28*, 622–629. [CrossRef]
10. Donehower, L.A.; Harvey, M.; Slagle, B.L.; McArthur, M.J.; Montgomery, C.A.; Butel, J.S.; Bradley, A. Mice deficient for p53 are developmentally normal but susceptible to spontaneous tumours. *Nature* **1992**, *356*, 215–221. [CrossRef]
11. Li, F.P.; Fraumeni, J.F. Rhabdomyosarcoma in children: Epidemiologic study and identification of a familial cancer syndrome. *J. Natl. Cancer Inst.* **1969**, *43*, 1365–1373. [PubMed]
12. Li, F.P.; Fraumeni, J.F. Soft-tissue sarcomas, breast cancer, and other neoplasms. A familial syndrome? *Ann. Intern. Med.* **1969**, *71*, 747–752. [CrossRef] [PubMed]
13. Srivastava, S.; Zou, Z.Q.; Pirollo, K.; Blattner, W.; Chang, E.H. Germ-line transmission of a mutated p53 gene in a cancer-prone family with Li-Fraumeni syndrome. *Nature* **1990**, *348*, 747–749. [CrossRef] [PubMed]
14. Malkin, D.; Li, F.P.; Strong, L.C.; Fraumeni, J.F.; Nelson, C.E.; Kim, D.H.; Kassel, J.; Gryka, M.A.; Bischoff, F.Z.; Tainsky, M.A.; et al. Germ line p53 mutations in a familial syndrome of breast cancer, sarcomas, and other neoplasms. *Science* **1990**, *250*, 1233–1238. [CrossRef]
15. Fields, S.; Jang, S.K. Presence of a potent transcription activating sequence in the p53 protein. *Science* **1990**, *249*, 1046–1049. [CrossRef] [PubMed]
16. Sullivan, K.D.; Galbraith, M.D.; Andrysik, Z.; Espinosa, J.M. Mechanisms of transcriptional regulation by p53. *Cell Death Differ.* **2018**, *25*, 133–143. [CrossRef]

17. Raycroft, L.; Wu, H.Y.; Lozano, G. Transcriptional activation by wild-type but not transforming mutants of the p53 anti-oncogene. *Science* **1990**, *249*, 1049–1051. [CrossRef]
18. Nishimura, M.; Arimura, Y.; Nozawa, K.; Kurumizaka, H. Linker DNA and histone contributions in nucleosome binding by p53. *J. Biochem.* **2020**, mvva081. [CrossRef]
19. Lang, Y.; Yu, C.; Tang, J.; Li, G.; Bai, R. Characterization of porcine p53 and its regulation by porcine Mdm2. *Gene* **2020**, *748*, 144699. [CrossRef]
20. Popova, G.; Ladds, M.J.G.W.; Johansson, L.; Saleh, A.; Larsson, J.; Sandberg, L.; Sahlberg, S.H.; Qian, W.; Gullberg, H.; Garg, N.; et al. Optimization of Tetrahydroindazoles as Inhibitors of Human Dihydroorotate Dehydrogenase and Evaluation of Their Activity and In Vitro Metabolic Stability. *J. Med. Chem.* **2020**, *63*, 3915–3934. [CrossRef]
21. Kurbegovic, A.; Trudel, M. The master regulators Myc and p53 cellular signaling and functions in polycystic kidney disease. *Cell. Signal.* **2020**, *71*, 109594. [CrossRef] [PubMed]
22. Patel, H.; Sheikh, M.S.; Huang, Y. ECRG2, a novel transcriptional target of p53, modulates cancer cell sensitivity to DNA damage. *Cell Death Dis.* **2020**, *11*, 543. [CrossRef] [PubMed]
23. Puzio-Kuter, A.M. The Role of p53 in Metabolic Regulation. *Genes Cancer* **2011**, *2*, 385–391. [CrossRef] [PubMed]
24. Muñoz-Fontela, C.; Mandinova, A.; Aaronson, S.A.; Lee, S.W. Emerging roles of p53 and other tumour-suppressor genes in immune regulation. *Nat. Rev. Immunol.* **2016**, *16*, 741–750. [CrossRef]
25. Kandoth, C.; McLellan, M.D.; Vandin, F.; Ye, K.; Niu, B.; Lu, C.; Xie, M.; Zhang, Q.; McMichael, J.F.; Wyczalkowski, M.A.; et al. Mutational landscape and significance across 12 major cancer types. *Nature* **2013**, *502*, 333–339. [CrossRef]
26. Kogan, S.; Carpizo, D. Pharmacological targeting of mutant p53. *Transl. Cancer Res.* **2016**, *5*, 698–706. [CrossRef]
27. Raghavan, V.; Agrahari, M.; Gowda, D.K. Virtual screening of p53 mutants reveals Y220S as an additional rescue drug target for PhiKan083 with higher binding characteristics. *Comput. Biol. Chem.* **2019**, *80*, 398–408. [CrossRef]
28. Li, X.; Zhang, X.-X.; Lin, Y.-X.; Xu, X.-M.; Li, L.; Yang, J.-B. Virtual Screening Based on Ensemble Docking Targeting Wild-Type p53 for Anticancer Drug Discovery. *Chem. Biodivers.* **2019**, *16*, e1900170. [CrossRef]
29. Synnott, N.C.; Bauer, M.R.; Madden, S.; Murray, A.; Klinger, R.; O'Donovan, N.; O'Connor, D.; Gallagher, W.M.; Crown, J.; Fersht, A.R.; et al. Mutant p53 as a therapeutic target for the treatment of triple-negative breast cancer: Preclinical investigation with the anti-p53 drug, PK11007. *Cancer Lett.* **2018**, *414*, 99–106. [CrossRef]
30. Multhoff, G.; Molls, M.; Radons, J. Chronic inflammation in cancer development. *Front. Immunol.* **2011**, *2*, 98. [CrossRef]
31. Kruk, J.; Aboul-Enein, H.Y. Reactive Oxygen and Nitrogen Species in Carcinogenesis: Implications of Oxidative Stress on the Progression and Development of Several Cancer Types. *Mini. Rev. Med. Chem.* **2017**, *17*, 904–919. [CrossRef]
32. Van Elsland, D.; Neefjes, J. Bacterial infections and cancer. *EMBO Rep.* **2018**, *19*, e46632. [CrossRef] [PubMed]
33. Uehara, I.; Tanaka, N. Role of p53 in the Regulation of the Inflammatory Tumor Microenvironment and Tumor Suppression. *Cancers* **2018**, *10*, 219. [CrossRef] [PubMed]
34. Okuda, Y.; Okuda, M.; Bernard, C.C.A. Regulatory role of p53 in experimental autoimmune encephalomyelitis. *J. Neuroimmunol.* **2003**, *135*, 29–37. [CrossRef]
35. Yamanishi, Y.; Boyle, D.L.; Pinkoski, M.J.; Mahboubi, A.; Lin, T.; Han, Z.; Zvaifler, N.J.; Green, D.R.; Firestein, G.S. Regulation of joint destruction and inflammation by p53 in collagen-induced arthritis. *Am. J. Pathol.* **2002**, *160*, 123–130. [CrossRef]
36. Davidson, L.A.; Callaway, E.S.; Kim, E.; Weeks, B.R.; Fan, Y.-Y.; Allred, C.D.; Chapkin, R.S. Targeted Deletion of p53 in Lgr5-Expressing Intestinal Stem Cells Promotes Colon Tumorigenesis in a Preclinical Model of Colitis-Associated Cancer. *Cancer Res.* **2015**, *75*, 5392–5397. [CrossRef]
37. Kawauchi, K.; Araki, K.; Tobiume, K.; Tanaka, N. Activated p53 induces NF-kappaB DNA binding but suppresses its transcriptional activation. *Biochem. Biophys. Res. Commun.* **2008**, *372*, 137–141. [CrossRef]
38. Son, D.-S.; Kabir, S.M.; Dong, Y.-L.; Lee, E.; Adunyah, S.E. Inhibitory effect of tumor suppressor p53 on proinflammatory chemokine expression in ovarian cancer cells by reducing proteasomal degradation of IκB. *PLoS ONE* **2012**, *7*, e51116. [CrossRef]

39. Blagih, J.; Buck, M.D.; Vousden, K.H. P53, cancer and the immune response. *J. Cell. Sci.* **2020**, *133*, jcs237453. [CrossRef]
40. Keates, S.; Hitti, Y.S.; Upton, M.; Kelly, C.P. Helicobacter pylori infection activates NF-kappa B in gastric epithelial cells. *Gastroenterology* **1997**, *113*, 1099–1109. [CrossRef]
41. Uemura, N.; Okamoto, S.; Yamamoto, S.; Matsumura, N.; Yamaguchi, S.; Yamakido, M.; Taniyama, K.; Sasaki, N.; Schlemper, R.J. Helicobacter pylori infection and the development of gastric cancer. *N. Engl. J. Med.* **2001**, *345*, 784–789. [CrossRef] [PubMed]
42. Matsumoto, Y.; Marusawa, H.; Kinoshita, K.; Endo, Y.; Kou, T.; Morisawa, T.; Azuma, T.; Okazaki, I.-M.; Honjo, T.; Chiba, T. Helicobacter pylori infection triggers aberrant expression of activation-induced cytidine deaminase in gastric epithelium. *Nat. Med.* **2007**, *13*, 470–476. [CrossRef] [PubMed]
43. Butin-Israeli, V.; Bui, T.M.; Wiesolek, H.L.; Mascarenhas, L.; Lee, J.J.; Mehl, L.C.; Knutson, K.R.; Adam, S.A.; Goldman, R.D.; Beyder, A.; et al. Neutrophil-induced genomic instability impedes resolution of inflammation and wound healing. *J. Clin. Invest.* **2019**, *129*, 712–726. [CrossRef] [PubMed]
44. Brazil, J.C.; Louis, N.A.; Parkos, C.A. The role of polymorphonuclear leukocyte trafficking in the perpetuation of inflammation during inflammatory bowel disease. *Inflamm. Bowel Dis.* **2013**, *19*, 1556–1565. [CrossRef] [PubMed]
45. Wieczorek, M.; Abualrous, E.T.; Sticht, J.; Álvaro-Benito, M.; Stolzenberg, S.; Noé, F.; Freund, C. Major Histocompatibility Complex (MHC) Class I and MHC Class II Proteins: Conformational Plasticity in Antigen Presentation. *Front. Immunol.* **2017**, *8*, 292. [CrossRef]
46. Griffioen, M.; Steegenga, W.T.; Ouwerkerk, I.J.; Peltenburg, L.T.; Jochemsen, A.G.; Schrier, P.I. Repression of the minimal HLA-B promoter by c-myc and p53 occurs through independent mechanisms. *Mol. Immunol.* **1998**, *35*, 829–835. [CrossRef]
47. Wang, B.; Niu, D.; Lai, L.; Ren, E.C. P53 increases MHC class I expression by upregulating the endoplasmic reticulum aminopeptidase ERAP1. *Nat. Commun.* **2013**, *4*, 2359. [CrossRef]
48. Zhu, K.; Wang, J.; Zhu, J.; Jiang, J.; Shou, J.; Chen, X. P53 induces TAP1 and enhances the transport of MHC class I peptides. *Oncogene* **1999**, *18*, 7740–7747. [CrossRef]
49. Garancher, A.; Suzuki, H.; Haricharan, S.; Chau, L.Q.; Masihi, M.B.; Rusert, J.M.; Norris, P.S.; Carrette, F.; Romero, M.M.; Morrissy, S.A.; et al. Tumor necrosis factor overcomes immune evasion in p53-mutant medulloblastoma. *Nat. Neurosci.* **2020**, *23*, 842–853. [CrossRef]
50. Sharpe, A.H.; Pauken, K.E. The diverse functions of the PD1 inhibitory pathway. *Nat. Rev. Immunol.* **2018**, *18*, 153–167. [CrossRef]
51. Freeman, G.J.; Long, A.J.; Iwai, Y.; Bourque, K.; Chernova, T.; Nishimura, H.; Fitz, L.J.; Malenkovich, N.; Okazaki, T.; Byrne, M.C.; et al. Engagement of the PD-1 immunoinhibitory receptor by a novel B7 family member leads to negative regulation of lymphocyte activation. *J. Exp. Med.* **2000**, *192*, 1027–1034. [CrossRef]
52. Cortez, M.A.; Ivan, C.; Valdecanas, D.; Wang, X.; Peltier, H.J.; Ye, Y.; Araujo, L.; Carbone, D.P.; Shilo, K.; Giri, D.K.; et al. PDL1 Regulation by p53 via miR-34. *J. Natl. Cancer Inst.* **2016**, *108*, djv303. [CrossRef] [PubMed]
53. Chamoto, K.; Hatae, R.; Honjo, T. Current issues and perspectives in PD-1 blockade cancer immunotherapy. *Int. J. Clin. Oncol.* **2020**, *25*, 790–800. [CrossRef] [PubMed]
54. Nie, L.; Cai, S.-Y.; Shao, J.-Z.; Chen, J. Toll-Like Receptors, Associated Biological Roles, and Signaling Networks in Non-Mammals. *Front. Immunol.* **2018**, *9*, 1523. [CrossRef] [PubMed]
55. Urban-Wojciuk, Z.; Khan, M.M.; Oyler, B.L.; Fåhraeus, R.; Marek-Trzonkowska, N.; Nita-Lazar, A.; Hupp, T.R.; Goodlett, D.R. The Role of TLRs in Anti-cancer Immunity and Tumor Rejection. *Front. Immunol.* **2019**, *10*, 2388. [CrossRef]
56. Menendez, D.; Lowe, J.M.; Snipe, J.; Resnick, M.A. Ligand dependent restoration of human TLR3 signaling and death in p53 mutant cells. *Oncotarget* **2016**, *7*, 61630–61642. [CrossRef]
57. Shatz, M.; Shats, I.; Menendez, D.; Resnick, M.A. P53 amplifies Toll-like receptor 5 response in human primary and cancer cells through interaction with multiple signal transduction pathways. *Oncotarget* **2015**, *6*, 16963–16980. [CrossRef]
58. Haricharan, S.; Brown, P. TLR4 has a TP53-dependent dual role in regulating breast cancer cell growth. *Proc. Natl. Acad. Sci. USA* **2015**, *112*, E3216–E3225. [CrossRef]

59. Menendez, D.; Snipe, J.; Marzec, J.; Innes, C.L.; Polack, F.P.; Caballero, M.T.; Schurman, S.H.; Kleeberger, S.R.; Resnick, M.A. P53-responsive TLR8 SNP enhances human innate immune response to respiratory syncytial virus. *J. Clin. Invest.* **2019**, *129*, 4875–4884. [CrossRef]
60. Rusanen, P.; Marttila, E.; Uittamo, J.; Hagström, J.; Salo, T.; Rautemaa-Richardson, R. TLR1-10, NF-κB and p53 expression is increased in oral lichenoid disease. *PLoS ONE* **2017**, *12*, e0181361. [CrossRef]
61. Zhang, Y.; Xia, G.; Zhang, Y.; Liu, J.; Liu, X.; Li, W.; Lv, Y.; Wei, S.; Liu, J.; Quan, J. Palmitate induces VSMC apoptosis via toll like receptor (TLR)4/ROS/p53 pathway. *Atherosclerosis* **2017**, *263*, 74–81. [CrossRef] [PubMed]
62. Huang, S.-W.; Chang, S.-H.; Mu, S.-W.; Jiang, H.-Y.; Wang, S.-T.; Kao, J.-K.; Huang, J.-L.; Wu, C.-Y.; Chen, Y.-J.; Shieh, J.-J. Imiquimod activates p53-dependent apoptosis in a human basal cell carcinoma cell line. *J. Dermatol. Sci.* **2016**, *81*, 182–191. [CrossRef] [PubMed]
63. Wellenstein, M.D.; Coffelt, S.B.; Duits, D.E.M.; Van Miltenburg, M.H.; Slagter, M.; De Rink, I.; Henneman, L.; Kas, S.M.; Prekovic, S.; Hau, C.-S.; et al. Loss of p53 triggers WNT-dependent systemic inflammation to drive breast cancer metastasis. *Nature* **2019**, *572*, 538–542. [CrossRef] [PubMed]
64. Bezzi, M.; Seitzer, N.; Ishikawa, T.; Reschke, M.; Chen, M.; Wang, G.; Mitchell, C.; Ng, C.; Katon, J.; Lunardi, A.; et al. Diverse genetic-driven immune landscapes dictate tumor progression through distinct mechanisms. *Nat. Med.* **2018**, *24*, 165–175. [CrossRef] [PubMed]
65. Walton, J.; Blagih, J.; Ennis, D.; Leung, E.; Dowson, S.; Farquharson, M.; Tookman, L.A.; Orange, C.; Athineos, D.; Mason, S.; et al. CRISPR/Cas9-Mediated Trp53 and Brca2 Knockout to Generate Improved Murine Models of Ovarian High-Grade Serous Carcinoma. *Cancer Res.* **2016**, *76*, 6118–6129. [CrossRef] [PubMed]
66. Ruddell, A.; Kelly-Spratt, K.S.; Furuya, M.; Parghi, S.S.; Kemp, C.J. P19/Arf and p53 suppress sentinel lymph node lymphangiogenesis and carcinoma metastasis. *Oncogene* **2008**, *27*, 3145–3155. [CrossRef] [PubMed]
67. Blagih, J.; Zani, F.; Chakravarty, P.; Hennequart, M.; Pilley, S.; Hobor, S.; Hock, A.K.; Walton, J.B.; Morton, J.P.; Gronroos, E.; et al. Cancer-Specific Loss of p53 Leads to a Modulation of Myeloid and T Cell Responses. *Cell Rep.* **2020**, *30*, 481–496. [CrossRef]
68. Li, D.; Bentley, C.; Anderson, A.; Wiblin, S.; Cleary, K.L.S.; Koustoulidou, S.; Hassanali, T.; Yates, J.; Greig, J.; Nordkamp, M.O.; et al. Development of a T-cell Receptor Mimic Antibody against Wild-Type p53 for Cancer Immunotherapy. *Cancer Res.* **2017**, *77*, 2699–2711. [CrossRef]
69. Low, L.; Goh, A.; Koh, J.; Lim, S.; Wang, C.-I. Targeting mutant p53-expressing tumours with a T cell receptor-like antibody specific for a wild-type antigen. *Nat. Commun.* **2019**, *10*, 5382. [CrossRef]
70. Kortylewski, M.; Yu, H. Stat3 as a Potential Target for Cancer Immunotherapy. *J. Immunother.* **2007**, *30*, 131–139. [CrossRef]
71. Wörmann, S.M.; Song, L.; Ai, J.; Diakopoulos, K.N.; Kurkowski, M.U.; Görgülü, K.; Ruess, D.; Campbell, A.; Doglioni, C.; Jodrell, D.; et al. Loss of P53 Function Activates JAK2-STAT3 Signaling to Promote Pancreatic Tumor Growth, Stroma Modification, and Gemcitabine Resistance in Mice and Is Associated With Patient Survival. *Gastroenterology* **2016**, *151*, 180–193. [CrossRef] [PubMed]
72. Nowak, D.G.; Cho, H.; Herzka, T.; Watrud, K.; DeMarco, D.V.; Wang, V.M.Y.; Senturk, S.; Fellmann, C.; Ding, D.; Beinortas, T.; et al. MYC Drives Pten/Trp53-Deficient Proliferation and Metastasis due to IL6 Secretion and AKT Suppression via PHLPP2. *Cancer Discov.* **2015**, *5*, 636–651. [CrossRef]
73. Calabrese, V.; Mallette, F.A.; Deschênes-Simard, X.; Ramanathan, S.; Gagnon, J.; Moores, A.; Ilangumaran, S.; Ferbeyre, G. SOCS1 links cytokine signaling to p53 and senescence. *Mol. Cell* **2009**, *36*, 754–767. [CrossRef] [PubMed]
74. Cooks, T.; Pateras, I.S.; Tarcic, O.; Solomon, H.; Schetter, A.J.; Wilder, S.; Lozano, G.; Pikarsky, E.; Forshew, T.; Rosenfeld, N.; et al. Mutant p53 prolongs NF-κB activation and promotes chronic inflammation and inflammation-associated colorectal cancer. *Cancer Cell* **2013**, *23*, 634–646. [CrossRef]
75. Rahnamoun, H.; Lu, H.; Duttke, S.H.; Benner, C.; Glass, C.K.; Lauberth, S.M. Mutant p53 shapes the enhancer landscape of cancer cells in response to chronic immune signaling. *Nat. Commun.* **2017**, *8*, 754. [CrossRef]
76. Ubertini, V.; Norelli, G.; D'Arcangelo, D.; Gurtner, A.; Cesareo, E.; Baldari, S.; Gentileschi, M.P.; Piaggio, G.; Nisticò, P.; Soddu, S.; et al. Mutant p53 gains new function in promoting inflammatory signals by repression of the secreted interleukin-1 receptor antagonist. *Oncogene* **2015**, *34*, 2493–2504. [CrossRef]
77. Headland, S.E.; Norling, L.V. The resolution of inflammation: Principles and challenges. *Semin. Immunol.* **2015**, *27*, 149–160. [CrossRef]

78. Singh, N.; Baby, D.; Rajguru, J.; Patil, P.; Thakkannavar, S.; Pujari, V. Inflammation and cancer. *Ann. Afr. Med.* **2019**, *18*, 121. [CrossRef] [PubMed]
79. Nathan, C.; Ding, A. Nonresolving Inflammation. *Cell* **2010**, *140*, 871–882. [CrossRef] [PubMed]
80. Chen, L.; Deng, H.; Cui, H.; Fang, J.; Zuo, Z.; Deng, J.; Li, Y.; Wang, X.; Zhao, L. Inflammatory responses and inflammation-associated diseases in organs. *Oncotarget* **2018**, *9*, 7204–7218. [CrossRef] [PubMed]
81. Kamp, D.W.; Shacter, E.; Weitzman, S.A. Chronic inflammation and cancer: The role of the mitochondria. *Oncology (Williston Park, N.Y.)* **2011**, *25*, 400–410, 413.
82. Maeda, H.; Akaike, T. Nitric oxide and oxygen radicals in infection, inflammation, and cancer. *Biochem. Mosc.* **1998**, *63*, 854–865.
83. Kawanishi, S.; Ohnishi, S.; Ma, N.; Hiraku, Y.; Oikawa, S.; Murata, M. Nitrative and oxidative DNA damage in infection-related carcinogenesis in relation to cancer stem cells. *Genes Environ.* **2016**, *38*, 26. [CrossRef] [PubMed]
84. Souici, A.-C. Transition mutation in codon 248 of the p53 tumor suppressor gene induced by reactive oxygen species and a nitric oxide-releasing compound. *Carcinogenesis* **2000**, *21*, 281–287. [CrossRef] [PubMed]
85. Coussens, L.M.; Werb, Z. Inflammation and cancer. *Nature* **2002**, *420*, 860–867. [CrossRef]
86. Varki, A.; Schnaar, R.L.; Crocker, P.R. I-Type Lectins. In *Essentials of Glycobiology*; Varki, A., Cummings, R.D., Esko, J.D., Stanley, P., Hart, G.W., Aebi, M., Darvill, A.G., Kinoshita, T., Packer, N.H., Prestegard, J.H., et al., Eds.; Cold Spring Harbor Laboratory Press: Cold Spring Harbor, NY, USA, 2015.
87. Siddiqui, S.S.; Matar, R.; Merheb, M.; Hodeify, R.; Vazhappilly, C.G.; Marton, J.; Shamsuddin, S.A.; Al Zouabi, H. Siglecs in Brain Function and Neurological Disorders. *Cells* **2019**, *8*, 1125. [CrossRef]
88. Siddiqui, S.; Schwarz, F.; Springer, S.; Khedri, Z.; Yu, H.; Deng, L.; Verhagen, A.; Naito-Matsui, Y.; Jiang, W.; Kim, D.; et al. Studies on the Detection, Expression, Glycosylation, Dimerization, and Ligand Binding Properties of Mouse Siglec-E. *J. Biol. Chem.* **2017**, *292*, 1029–1037. [CrossRef]
89. Siddiqui, S.S.; Springer, S.A.; Verhagen, A.; Sundaramurthy, V.; Alisson-Silva, F.; Jiang, W.; Ghosh, P.; Varki, A. The Alzheimer's disease-protective CD33 splice variant mediates adaptive loss of function via diversion to an intracellular pool. *J. Biol. Chem.* **2017**, *292*, 15312–15320. [CrossRef]
90. Läubli, H.; Pearce, O.M.T.; Schwarz, F.; Siddiqui, S.S.; Deng, L.; Stanczak, M.A.; Deng, L.; Verhagen, A.; Secrest, P.; Lusk, C.; et al. Engagement of myelomonocytic Siglecs by tumor-associated ligands modulates the innate immune response to cancer. *Proc. Natl. Acad. Sci. USA* **2014**, *111*, 14211–14216. [CrossRef]
91. Läubli, H.; Alisson-Silva, F.; Stanczak, M.A.; Siddiqui, S.S.; Deng, L.; Verhagen, A.; Varki, N.; Varki, A. Lectin galactoside-binding soluble 3 binding protein (LGALS3BP) is a tumor-associated immunomodulatory ligand for CD33-related Siglecs. *J. Biol. Chem.* **2014**, *289*, 33481–33491. [CrossRef]
92. Stanczak, M.A.; Siddiqui, S.S.; Trefny, M.P.; Thommen, D.S.; Boligan, K.F.; Von Gunten, S.; Tzankov, A.; Tietze, L.; Lardinois, D.; Heinzelmann-Schwarz, V.; et al. Self-associated molecular patterns mediate cancer immune evasion by engaging Siglecs on T cells. *J. Clin. Invest.* **2018**, *128*, 4912–4923. [CrossRef] [PubMed]
93. Uchiyama, S.; Sun, J.; Fukahori, K.; Ando, N.; Wu, M.; Schwarz, F.; Siddiqui, S.S.; Varki, A.; Marth, J.D.; Nizet, V. Dual actions of group B Streptococcus capsular sialic acid provide resistance to platelet-mediated antimicrobial killing. *Proc. Natl. Acad. Sci. USA* **2019**, *116*, 7465–7470. [CrossRef] [PubMed]
94. Saha, S.; Siddiqui, S.S.; Khan, N.; Verhagen, A.; Jiang, W.; Springer, S.; Ghosh, P.; Varki, A. Controversies about the subcellular localization and mechanisms of action of the Alzheimer's disease-protective CD33 splice variant. *Acta Neuropathol.* **2019**, *138*, 671–672. [CrossRef]
95. Schwarz, F.; Landig, C.S.; Siddiqui, S.; Secundino, I.; Olson, J.; Varki, N.; Nizet, V.; Varki, A. Paired Siglec receptors generate opposite inflammatory responses to a human-specific pathogen. *EMBO J.* **2017**, *36*, 751–760. [CrossRef] [PubMed]
96. De la Vega, M.R.; Chapman, E.; Zhang, D.D. NRF2 and the Hallmarks of Cancer. *Cancer Cell* **2018**, *34*, 21–43. [CrossRef] [PubMed]
97. Wu, S.; Lu, H.; Bai, Y. Nrf2 in cancers: A double-edged sword. *Cancer Med.* **2019**, *8*, 2252–2267. [CrossRef]
98. Ahmed, S.M.U.; Luo, L.; Namani, A.; Wang, X.J.; Tang, X. Nrf2 signaling pathway: Pivotal roles in inflammation. *Biochim. et Biophys. Acta (BBA) Mol. Basis Dis.* **2017**, *1863*, 585–597. [CrossRef]
99. Tu, W.; Wang, H.; Li, S.; Liu, Q.; Sha, H. The Anti-Inflammatory and Anti-Oxidant Mechanisms of the Keap1/Nrf2/ARE Signaling Pathway in Chronic Diseases. *Aging Dis.* **2019**, *10*, 637. [CrossRef]

100. Chen, W.; Sun, Z.; Wang, X.-J.; Jiang, T.; Huang, Z.; Fang, D.; Zhang, D.D. Direct Interaction between Nrf2 and p21Cip1/WAF1 Upregulates the Nrf2-Mediated Antioxidant Response. *Mol. Cell* **2009**, *34*, 663–673. [CrossRef]
101. Zimta, A.-A.; Cenariu, D.; Irimie, A.; Magdo, L.; Nabavi, S.M.; Atanasov, A.G.; Berindan-Neagoe, I. The Role of Nrf2 Activity in Cancer Development and Progression. *Cancers* **2019**, *11*, 1755. [CrossRef]
102. Menegon, S.; Columbano, A.; Giordano, S. The Dual Roles of NRF2 in Cancer. *Trends Mol. Med.* **2016**, *22*, 578–593. [CrossRef] [PubMed]
103. Jaramillo, M.C.; Zhang, D.D. The emerging role of the Nrf2-Keap1 signaling pathway in cancer. *Genes Dev.* **2013**, *27*, 2179–2191. [CrossRef]
104. Hussain, T.; Tan, B.; Yin, Y.; Blachier, F.; Tossou, M.C.B.; Rahu, N. Oxidative Stress and Inflammation: What Polyphenols Can Do for Us? *Oxid. Med. Cell. Longev.* **2016**, *2016*, 1–9. [CrossRef] [PubMed]
105. Redza-Dutordoir, M.; Averill-Bates, D.A. Activation of apoptosis signalling pathways by reactive oxygen species. *Biochim. et Biophys. Acta (BBA) Mol. Cell Res.* **2016**, *1863*, 2977–2992. [CrossRef] [PubMed]
106. Chen, M.; Chen, X.; Song, X.; Muhammad, A.; Jia, R.; Zou, Y.; Yin, L.; Li, L.; He, C.; Ye, G.; et al. The immune-adjuvant activity and the mechanism of resveratrol on pseudorabies virus vaccine in a mouse model. *Int. Immunopharmacol.* **2019**, *76*, 105876. [CrossRef] [PubMed]
107. Sun, X.; Jia, H.; Xu, Q.; Zhao, C.; Xu, C. Lycopene alleviates H_2O_2-induced oxidative stress, inflammation and apoptosis in bovine mammary epithelial cells via the NFE2L2 signaling pathway. *Food Funct.* **2019**, *10*, 6276–6285. [CrossRef] [PubMed]
108. Nadeem, A.; Ahmad, S.F.; Al-Harbi, N.O.; Attia, S.M.; Alshammari, M.A.; Alzahrani, K.S.; Bakheet, S.A. Increased oxidative stress in the cerebellum and peripheral immune cells leads to exaggerated autism-like repetitive behavior due to deficiency of antioxidant response in BTBR T + tf/J mice. *Prog. Neuropsychopharmacol. Biol. Psychiatry* **2019**, *89*, 245–253. [CrossRef]
109. Solleiro-Villavicencio, H.; Rivas-Arancibia, S. Effect of Chronic Oxidative Stress on Neuroinflammatory Response Mediated by CD4+T Cells in Neurodegenerative Diseases. *Front. Cell. Neurosci.* **2018**, *12*, 114. [CrossRef]
110. Karin, M. NF-B as a Critical Link Between Inflammation and Cancer. *Cold Spring Harb. Perspect. Biol.* **2009**, *1*, a000141. [CrossRef]
111. Plewka, D.; Plewka, A.; Miskiewicz, A.; Morek, M.; Bogunia, E. Nuclear factor-kappa B as potential therapeutic target in human colon cancer. *J. Cancer Res. Ther.* **2018**, *14*, 516. [CrossRef]
112. Chen, J. The Cell-Cycle Arrest and Apoptotic Functions of p53 in Tumor Initiation and Progression. *Cold Spring Harb. Perspect. Med.* **2016**, *6*, a026104. [CrossRef] [PubMed]
113. Cordani, M.; Butera, G.; Pacchiana, R.; Masetto, F.; Mullappilly, N.; Riganti, C.; Donadelli, M. Mutant p53-Associated Molecular Mechanisms of ROS Regulation in Cancer Cells. *Biomolecules* **2020**, *10*, 361. [CrossRef] [PubMed]
114. Chen, Y.; Liu, K.; Shi, Y.; Shao, C. The tango of ROS and p53 in tissue stem cells. *Cell Death Differ.* **2018**, *25*, 639–641. [CrossRef]
115. Olivos, D.; Mayo, L. Emerging Non-Canonical Functions and Regulation by p53: P53 and Stemness. *Int. J. Mol. Sci.* **2016**, *17*, 1982. [CrossRef] [PubMed]
116. Reuter, S.; Gupta, S.C.; Chaturvedi, M.M.; Aggarwal, B.B. Oxidative stress, inflammation, and cancer: How are they linked? *Free Radic. Biol. Med.* **2010**, *49*, 1603–1616. [CrossRef] [PubMed]
117. Fernando, W.; Rupasinghe, H.P.V.; Hoskin, D.W. Dietary phytochemicals with anti-oxidant and pro-oxidant activities: A double-edged sword in relation to adjuvant chemotherapy and radiotherapy? *Cancer Lett.* **2019**, *452*, 168–177. [CrossRef]
118. Wu, Y.; Lee, S.; Bobadilla, S.; Duan, S.Z.; Liu, X. High glucose-induced p53 phosphorylation contributes to impairment of endothelial antioxidant system. *Biochim. et Biophys. Acta (BBA) Mol. Basis Dis.* **2017**, *1863*, 2355–2362. [CrossRef]
119. D'Angelo, S.; Martino, E.; Ilisso, C.P.; Bagarolo, M.L.; Porcelli, M.; Cacciapuoti, G. Pro-oxidant and pro-apoptotic activity of polyphenol extract from Annurca apple and its underlying mechanisms in human breast cancer cells. *Int. J. Oncol.* **2017**, *51*, 939–948. [CrossRef]
120. Sablina, A.A.; Budanov, A.V.; Ilyinskaya, G.V.; Agapova, L.S.; Kravchenko, J.E.; Chumakov, P.M. The antioxidant function of the p53 tumor suppressor. *Nat. Med.* **2005**, *11*, 1306–1313. [CrossRef]

121. Vazhappilly, C.G.; Ansari, S.A.; Al-Jaleeli, R.; Al-Azawi, A.M.; Ramadan, W.S.; Menon, V.; Hodeify, R.; Siddiqui, S.S.; Merheb, M.; Matar, R.; et al. Role of flavonoids in thrombotic, cardiovascular, and inflammatory diseases. *Inflammopharmacol* **2019**, *27*, 863–869. [CrossRef]
122. Gunathilake, K.; Ranaweera, K.; Rupasinghe, H. In Vitro Anti-Inflammatory Properties of Selected Green Leafy Vegetables. *Biomedicines* **2018**, *6*, 107. [CrossRef] [PubMed]
123. George, V.C.; Vijesh, V.V.; Amararathna, D.I.M.; Lakshmi, C.A.; Anbarasu, K.; Kumar, D.R.N.; Ethiraj, K.R.; Kumar, R.A.; Rupasinghe, H.P.V. Mechanism of Action of Flavonoids in Prevention of Inflammation-Associated Skin Cancer. *CMC* **2016**, *23*, 3697–3716. [CrossRef] [PubMed]
124. Spiegel, M.; Andruniów, T.; Sroka, Z. Flavones' and Flavonols' Antiradical Structure–Activity Relationship—A Quantum Chemical Study. *Antioxidants* **2020**, *9*, 461. [CrossRef] [PubMed]
125. Sarian, M.N.; Ahmed, Q.U.; Mat So'ad, S.Z.; Alhassan, A.M.; Murugesu, S.; Perumal, V.; Syed Mohamad, S.N.A.; Khatib, A.; Latip, J. Antioxidant and Antidiabetic Effects of Flavonoids: A Structure-Activity Relationship Based Study. *BioMed Res. Int.* **2017**, *2017*, 8386065. [CrossRef] [PubMed]
126. Sordon, S.; Popłoński, J.; Milczarek, M.; Stachowicz, M.; Tronina, T.; Kucharska, A.Z.; Wietrzyk, J.; Huszcza, E. Structure–Antioxidant–Antiproliferative Activity Relationships of Natural C7 and C7–C8 Hydroxylated Flavones and Flavanones. *Antioxidants* **2019**, *8*, 210. [CrossRef]
127. Murakami, A.; Ashida, H.; Terao, J. Multitargeted cancer prevention by quercetin. *Cancer Lett.* **2008**, *269*, 315–325. [CrossRef]
128. Zhu, Q.; Liu, M.; He, Y.; Yang, B. Quercetin protect cigarette smoke extracts induced inflammation and apoptosis in RPE cells. *Artif. Cells Nanomed. Biotechnol.* **2019**, *47*, 2010–2015. [CrossRef]
129. Lisek, K.; Campaner, E.; Ciani, Y.; Walerych, D.; Del Sal, G. Mutant p53 tunes the NRF2-dependent antioxidant response to support survival of cancer cells. *Oncotarget* **2018**, *9*, 20508–20523. [CrossRef]
130. Han, C.; Sun, T.; Xv, G.; Wang, S.; Gu, J.; Liu, C. Berberine ameliorates CCl4-induced liver injury in rats through regulation of the Nrf2-Keap1-ARE and p53 signaling pathways. *Mol. Med. Rep.* **2019**, *20*, 3095–3102. [CrossRef]
131. Das, L.; Vinayak, M. Long Term Effect of Curcumin in Restoration of Tumour Suppressor p53 and Phase-II Antioxidant Enzymes via Activation of Nrf2 Signalling and Modulation of Inflammation in Prevention of Cancer. *PLoS ONE* **2015**, *10*, e0124000. [CrossRef]
132. Zhang, S.; Qi, Y.; Xu, Y.; Han, X.; Peng, J.; Liu, K.; Sun, C.K. Protective effect of flavonoid-rich extract from Rosa laevigata Michx on cerebral ischemia–reperfusion injury through suppression of apoptosis and inflammation. *Neurochem. Int.* **2013**, *63*, 522–532. [CrossRef]
133. Ahmed, O.M.; Ahmed, A.A.; Fahim, H.I.; Zaky, M.Y. Quercetin and naringenin abate diethylnitrosamine/acetylaminofluorene-induced hepatocarcinogenesis in Wistar rats: The roles of oxidative stress, inflammation and cell apoptosis. *Drug Chem. Toxicol.* **2019**, 1–12. [CrossRef]
134. Le, N.H.; Kim, C.-S.; Park, T.; Park, J.H.Y.; Sung, M.-K.; Lee, D.G.; Hong, S.-M.; Choe, S.-Y.; Goto, T.; Kawada, T.; et al. Quercetin Protects against Obesity-Induced Skeletal Muscle Inflammation and Atrophy. *Mediat. Inflamm.* **2014**, *2014*, 834294. [CrossRef]
135. Perdicaro, D.J.; Rodriguez Lanzi, C.; Gambarte Tudela, J.; Miatello, R.M.; Oteiza, P.I.; Vazquez Prieto, M.A. Quercetin attenuates adipose hypertrophy, in part through activation of adipogenesis in rats fed a high-fat diet. *J. Nutr. Biochem.* **2020**, *79*, 108352. [CrossRef] [PubMed]
136. Min, K.; Ebeler, S.E. Quercetin inhibits hydrogen peroxide-induced DNA damage and enhances DNA repair in Caco-2 cells. *Food Chem. Toxicol.* **2009**, *47*, 2716–2722. [CrossRef] [PubMed]
137. Wang, X.; Li, H.; Wang, H.; Shi, J. Quercetin attenuates high glucose-induced injury in human retinal pigment epithelial cell line ARPE-19 by up-regulation of miR-29b. *J. Biochem.* **2020**, *167*, 495–502. [CrossRef] [PubMed]
138. Darband, S.G.; Sadighparvar, S.; Yousefi, B.; Kaviani, M.; Ghaderi-Pakdel, F.; Mihanfar, A.; Rahimi, Y.; Mobaraki, K.; Majidinia, M. Quercetin attenuated oxidative DNA damage through NRF2 signaling pathway in rats with DMH induced colon carcinogenesis. *Life Sci.* **2020**, *253*, 117584. [CrossRef]
139. Clemente-Soto, A.; Salas-Vidal, E.; Milan-Pacheco, C.; Sánchez-Carranza, J.; Peralta-Zaragoza, O.; González-Maya, L. Quercetin induces G2 phase arrest and apoptosis with the activation of p53 in an E6 expression-independent manner in HPV-positive human cervical cancer-derived cells. *Mol. Med. Rep.* **2019**, *19*, 2097–2106. [CrossRef]
140. Neuwirthová, J.; Gál, B.; Smilek, P.; Urbánková, P. Potential of the Flavonoid Quercetin to Prevent and Treat Cancer—Current Status of Research. *Klin. Onkol.* **2018**, *31*, 184–190. [CrossRef]

141. Guo, Y.; Xu, N.; Sun, W.; Zhao, Y.; Li, C.; Guo, M. Luteolin reduces inflammation in *Staphylococcus aureus*-induced mastitis by inhibiting NF-κB activation and MMPs expression. *Oncotarget* **2017**, *8*, 28481–28493. [CrossRef]
142. AL-Megrin, W.A.; Alomar, S.; Alkhuriji, A.F.; Metwally, D.M.; Mohamed, S.K.; Kassab, R.B.; Abdel Moneim, A.E.; El-Khadragy, M.F. Luteolin protects against testicular injury induced by lead acetate by activating the Nrf2/ HO^{-1} pathway. *IUBMB Life* **2020**, *72*, 1787–1798. [CrossRef]
143. Lin, Y.; Shi, R.; Wang, X.; Shen, H.-M. Luteolin, a flavonoid with potential for cancer prevention and therapy. *Curr. Cancer Drug Targets* **2008**, *8*, 634–646. [CrossRef] [PubMed]
144. Wang, X.; Yuan, T.; Yin, N.; Ma, X.; Zhang, Z.; Zhu, Z.; Shaukat, A.; Deng, G. Luteoloside Protects the Uterus from Staphylococcus aureus-Induced Inflammation, Apoptosis, and Injury. *Inflammation* **2018**, *41*, 1702–1716. [CrossRef] [PubMed]
145. Li, L.; Luo, W.; Qian, Y.; Zhu, W.; Qian, J.; Li, J.; Jin, Y.; Xu, X.; Liang, G. Luteolin protects against diabetic cardiomyopathy by inhibiting NF-κB-mediated inflammation and activating the Nrf2-mediated antioxidant responses. *Phytomedicine* **2019**, *59*, 152774. [CrossRef] [PubMed]
146. Amin, A.R.M.R.; Wang, D.; Zhang, H.; Peng, S.; Shin, H.J.C.; Brandes, J.C.; Tighiouart, M.; Khuri, F.R.; Chen, Z.G.; Shin, D.M. Enhanced Anti-tumor Activity by the Combination of the Natural Compounds (−)-Epigallocatechin-3-gallate and Luteolin: Potential Role of p53. *J. Biol. Chem.* **2010**, *285*, 34557–34565. [CrossRef]
147. Dai, C.-Q.; Luo, T.-T.; Luo, S.-C.; Wang, J.-Q.; Wang, S.-M.; Bai, Y.-H.; Yang, Y.-L.; Wang, Y.-Y. P53 and mitochondrial dysfunction: Novel insight of neurodegenerative diseases. *J. Bioenerg. Biomembr.* **2016**, *48*, 337–347. [CrossRef]
148. Jiang, Z.-Q.; Li, M.-H.; Qin, Y.-M.; Jiang, H.-Y.; Zhang, X.; Wu, M.H. Luteolin Inhibits Tumorigenesis and Induces Apoptosis of Non-Small Cell Lung Cancer Cells via Regulation of MicroRNA-34a-5p. *Int. J. Mol. Sci.* **2018**, *19*, 447. [CrossRef]
149. Pérez-Sánchez, A.; Barrajón-Catalán, E.; Herranz-López, M.; Castillo, J.; Micol, V. Lemon balm extract (Melissa officinalis, L.) promotes melanogenesis and prevents UVB-induced oxidative stress and DNA damage in a skin cell model. *J. Dermatol. Sci.* **2016**, *84*, 169–177. [CrossRef]
150. George, V.C.; Kumar, D.R.N.; Suresh, P.K.; Kumar, S.; Kumar, R.A. Comparative Studies to Evaluate Relative in vitro Potency of Luteolin in Inducing Cell Cycle Arrest and Apoptosis in HaCaT and A375 Cells. *Asian Pac. J. Cancer Prev.* **2013**, *14*, 631–637. [CrossRef]
151. Wang, T.-T.; Wang, S.-K.; Huang, G.-L.; Sun, G.-J. Luteolin Induced-growth Inhibition and Apoptosis of Human Esophageal Squamous Carcinoma Cell Line Eca109 Cells in vitro. *Asian Pac. J. Cancer Prev.* **2012**, *13*, 5455–5461. [CrossRef]
152. Wang, J.; Li, P.; Qin, T.; Sun, D.; Zhao, X.; Zhang, B. Protective effect of epigallocatechin-3-gallate against neuroinflammation and anxiety-like behavior in a rat model of myocardial infarction. *Brain Behav.* **2020**, *10*, e01633. [CrossRef] [PubMed]
153. Ren, J.L.; Yu, Q.X.; Liang, W.C.; Leung, P.Y.; Ng, T.K.; Chu, W.K.; Pang, C.P.; Chan, S.O. Green tea extract attenuates LPS-induced retinal inflammation in rats. *Sci. Rep.* **2018**, *8*, 429. [CrossRef] [PubMed]
154. Oblak, A.; Jerala, R. Toll-Like Receptor 4 Activation in Cancer Progression and Therapy. *Clin. Dev. Immunol.* **2011**, *2011*, 1–12. [CrossRef] [PubMed]
155. Chen, C.-Y.; Kao, C.-L.; Liu, C.-M. The Cancer Prevention, Anti-Inflammatory and Anti-Oxidation of Bioactive Phytochemicals Targeting the TLR4 Signaling Pathway. *Int. J. Mol. Sci.* **2018**, *19*, 2729. [CrossRef] [PubMed]
156. Shen, H.; Wu, N.; Liu, Z.; Zhao, H.; Zhao, M. Epigallocatechin-3-gallate alleviates paraquat-induced acute lung injury and inhibits upregulation of toll-like receptors. *Life Sci.* **2017**, *170*, 25–32. [CrossRef]
157. Al-Maghrebi, M.; Alnajem, A.S.; Esmaeil, A. Epigallocatechin-3-gallate modulates germ cell apoptosis through the SAFE/Nrf2 signaling pathway. *Naunyn Schmiedeberg's Arch. Pharmacol.* **2020**, *393*, 663–671. [CrossRef]
158. He, Y.; Tan, D.; Bai, B.; Wu, Z.; Ji, S. Epigallocatechin-3-gallate attenuates acrylamide-induced apoptosis and astrogliosis in rat cerebral cortex. *Toxicol. Mech. Methods* **2017**, *27*, 298–306. [CrossRef]
159. Remely, M.; Ferk, F.; Sterneder, S.; Setayesh, T.; Roth, S.; Kepcija, T.; Noorizadeh, R.; Rebhan, I.; Greunz, M.; Beckmann, J.; et al. EGCG Prevents High Fat Diet-Induced Changes in Gut Microbiota, Decreases of DNA Strand Breaks, and Changes in Expression and DNA Methylation of *Dnmt1* and *MLH1* in C57BL/6J Male Mice. *Oxid. Med. Cell. Longev.* **2017**, *2017*, 3079148. [CrossRef]

160. George, V.C.; Dellaire, G.; Rupasinghe, H.P.V. Plant flavonoids in cancer chemoprevention: Role in genome stability. *J. Nutr. Biochem.* **2017**, *45*, 1–14. [CrossRef]
161. George, V.C.; Ansari, S.A.; Chelakkot, V.S.; Chelakkot, A.L.; Chelakkot, C.; Menon, V.; Ramadan, W.; Ethiraj, K.R.; El-Awady, R.; Mantso, T.; et al. DNA-dependent protein kinase: Epigenetic alterations and the role in genomic stability of cancer. *Mutat. Res. Rev. Mutat. Res.* **2019**, *780*, 92–105. [CrossRef]
162. De Silva, A.B.K.H.; Rupasinghe, H.P.V. Polyphenols composition and anti-diabetic properties in vitro of haskap (Lonicera caerulea L.) berries in relation to cultivar and harvesting date. *J. Food Compos. Anal.* **2020**, *88*, 103402. [CrossRef]
163. Gan, Y.; Fu, Y.; Yang, L.; Chen, J.; Lei, H.; Liu, Q. Cyanidin-3-O-Glucoside and Cyanidin Protect Against Intestinal Barrier Damage and 2,4,6-Trinitrobenzenesulfonic Acid-Induced Colitis. *J. Med. Food* **2020**, *23*, 90–99. [CrossRef] [PubMed]
164. Zheng, H.X.; Qi, S.S.; He, J.; Hu, C.Y.; Han, H.; Jiang, H.; Li, X.S. Cyanidin-3-glucoside from Black Rice Ameliorates Diabetic Nephropathy via Reducing Blood Glucose, Suppressing Oxidative Stress and Inflammation, and Regulating Transforming Growth Factor β1/Smad Expression. *J. Agric. Food Chem.* **2020**, *68*, 4399–4410. [CrossRef]
165. Liu, Z.; Hu, Y.; Li, X.; Mei, Z.; Wu, S.; He, Y.; Jiang, X.; Sun, J.; Xiao, J.; Deng, L.; et al. Nanoencapsulation of Cyanidin-3-O-glucoside Enhances Protection Against UVB-Induced Epidermal Damage through Regulation of p53-Mediated Apoptosis in Mice. *J. Agric. Food Chem.* **2018**, *66*, 5359–5367. [CrossRef] [PubMed]
166. Amararathna, M.; Hoskin, D.W.; Rupasinghe, H.P.V. Anthocyanin-rich haskap (Lonicera caerulea L.) berry extracts reduce nitrosamine-induced DNA damage in human normal lung epithelial cells. *Food Chem. Toxicol.* **2020**, *141*, 111404. [CrossRef] [PubMed]
167. Hu, Y.; Ma, Y.; Wu, S.; Chen, T.; He, Y.; Sun, J.; Jiao, R.; Jiang, X.; Huang, Y.; Deng, L.; et al. Protective Effect of Cyanidin-3-O-Glucoside against Ultraviolet B Radiation-Induced Cell Damage in Human HaCaT Keratinocytes. *Front. Pharmacol.* **2016**, *7*, 301. [CrossRef]
168. George, V.C.; Rupasinghe, H.P.V. Apple Flavonoids Suppress Carcinogen-Induced DNA Damage in Normal Human Bronchial Epithelial Cells. *Oxid. Med. Cell. Longev.* **2017**, *2017*, 1767198. [CrossRef]
169. Kaewmool, C.; Udomruk, S.; Phitak, T.; Pothacharoen, P.; Kongtawelert, P. Cyanidin-3-O-Glucoside Protects PC12 Cells Against Neuronal Apoptosis Mediated by LPS-Stimulated BV2 Microglial Activation. *Neurotox. Res.* **2020**, *37*, 111–125. [CrossRef]
170. Meng, H.; Fu, G.; Shen, J.; Shen, K.; Xu, Z.; Wang, Y.; Jin, B.; Pan, H. Ameliorative Effect of Daidzein on Cisplatin-Induced Nephrotoxicity in Mice via Modulation of Inflammation, Oxidative Stress, and Cell Death. *Oxid. Med. Cell. Longev.* **2017**, *2017*, 3140680. [CrossRef]
171. Sakamoto, Y.; Naka, A.; Ohara, N.; Kondo, K.; Iida, K. Daidzein regulates proinflammatory adipokines thereby improving obesity-related inflammation through PPARγ. *Mol. Nutr. Food Res.* **2014**, *58*, 718–726. [CrossRef]
172. Feng, G.; Sun, B.; Li, T. Daidzein attenuates lipopolysaccharide-induced acute lung injury via toll-like receptor 4/NF-kappaB pathway. *Int. Immunopharmacol.* **2015**, *26*, 392–400. [CrossRef] [PubMed]
173. Iovine, B.; Iannella, M.L.; Gasparri, F.; Monfrecola, G.; Bevilacqua, M.A. Synergic Effect of Genistein and Daidzein on UVB-Induced DNA Damage: An Effective Photoprotective Combination. *J. Biomed. Biotechnol.* **2011**, *2011*, 692846. [CrossRef] [PubMed]
174. Iovine, B.; Garofalo, M.; Orefice, M.; Giannini, V.; Gasparri, F.; Monfrecola, G.; Bevilacqua, M.A. Isoflavones in aglycone solution enhance ultraviolet B-induced DNA damage repair efficiency. *Clin. Exp. Dermatol.* **2014**, *39*, 391–394. [CrossRef] [PubMed]
175. Zare, M.F.R.; Rakhshan, K.; Aboutaleb, N.; Nikbakht, F.; Naderi, N.; Bakhshesh, M.; Azizi, Y. Apigenin attenuates doxorubicin induced cardiotoxicity via reducing oxidative stress and apoptosis in male rats. *Life Sci.* **2019**, *232*, 116623. [CrossRef]
176. Li, F.; Lang, F.; Zhang, H.; Xu, L.; Wang, Y.; Zhai, C.; Hao, E. Apigenin Alleviates Endotoxin-Induced Myocardial Toxicity by Modulating Inflammation, Oxidative Stress, and Autophagy. *Oxid. Med. Cell. Longev.* **2017**, *2017*, 2302896. [CrossRef] [PubMed]
177. Mirzoeva, S.; Tong, X.; Bridgeman, B.B.; Plebanek, M.P.; Volpert, O.V. Apigenin Inhibits UVB-Induced Skin Carcinogenesis: The Role of Thrombospondin-1 as an Anti-Inflammatory Factor. *Neoplasia* **2018**, *20*, 930–942. [CrossRef]

178. Ai, X.-Y.; Qin, Y.; Liu, H.-J.; Cui, Z.-H.; Li, M.; Yang, J.-H.; Zhong, W.-L.; Liu, Y.-R.; Chen, S.; Sun, T.; et al. Apigenin inhibits colonic inflammation and tumorigenesis by suppressing STAT3-NF-κB signaling. *Oncotarget* **2017**, *8*, 100216–100226. [CrossRef] [PubMed]
179. Thangaiyan, R.; Robert, B.M.; Arjunan, S.; Govindasamy, K.; Nagarajan, R.P. Preventive effect of apigenin against isoproterenol-induced apoptosis in cardiomyoblasts. *J. Biochem. Mol. Toxicol.* **2018**, *32*, e22213. [CrossRef]
180. Sarkaki, A.; Farbood, Y.; Mansouri, S.M.T.; Badavi, M.; Khorsandi, L.; Dehcheshmeh, M.G.; Shooshtari, M.K. Chrysin prevents cognitive and hippocampal long-term potentiation deficits and inflammation in rat with cerebral hypoperfusion and reperfusion injury. *Life Sci.* **2019**, *226*, 202–209. [CrossRef]
181. Li, T.-F.; Ma, J.; Han, X.-W.; Jia, Y.-X.; Yuan, H.-F.; Shui, S.-F.; Guo, D.; Yan, L. Chrysin ameliorates cerebral ischemia/reperfusion (I/R) injury in rats by regulating the PI3K/Akt/mTOR pathway. *Neurochem. Int.* **2019**, *129*, 104496. [CrossRef]
182. Del Fabbro, L.; Jesse, C.R.; De Gomes, M.G.; Borges Filho, C.; Donato, F.; Souza, L.C.; Goes, A.R.; Furian, A.F.; Boeira, S.P. The flavonoid chrysin protects against zearalenone induced reproductive toxicity in male mice. *Toxicon* **2019**, *165*, 13–21. [CrossRef] [PubMed]
183. El-Marasy, S.A.; El Awdan, S.A.; Abd-Elsalam, R.M. Protective role of chrysin on thioacetamide-induced hepatic encephalopathy in rats. *Chem. Biol. Interact.* **2019**, *299*, 111–119. [CrossRef] [PubMed]
184. Takaoka, O.; Mori, T.; Ito, F.; Okimura, H.; Kataoka, H.; Tanaka, Y.; Koshiba, A.; Kusuki, I.; Shigehiro, S.; Amami, T.; et al. Daidzein-rich isoflavone aglycones inhibit cell growth and inflammation in endometriosis. *J. Steroid Biochem. Mol. Biol.* **2018**, *181*, 125–132. [CrossRef] [PubMed]
185. Atiq, A.; Shal, B.; Naveed, M.; Khan, A.; Ali, J.; Zeeshan, S.; Al-Sharari, S.D.; Kim, Y.S.; Khan, S. Diadzein ameliorates 5-fluorouracil-induced intestinal mucositis by suppressing oxidative stress and inflammatory mediators in rodents. *Eur. J. Pharmacol.* **2019**, *843*, 292–306. [CrossRef]
186. Yoshida, H.; Watanabe, W.; Oomagari, H.; Tsuruta, E.; Shida, M.; Kurokawa, M. Citrus flavonoid naringenin inhibits TLR2 expression in adipocytes. *J. Nutr. Biochem.* **2013**, *24*, 1276–1284. [CrossRef]
187. Zhang, F.; Dong, W.; Zeng, W.; Zhang, L.; Zhang, C.; Qiu, Y.; Wang, L.; Yin, X.; Zhang, C.; Liang, W. Naringenin prevents TGF-β1 secretion from breast cancer and suppresses pulmonary metastasis by inhibiting PKC activation. *Breast Cancer Res.* **2016**, *18*, 38. [CrossRef]
188. Chtourou, Y.; Slima, A.B.; Makni, M.; Gdoura, R.; Fetoui, H. Naringenin protects cardiac hypercholesterolemia-induced oxidative stress and subsequent necroptosis in rats. *Pharmacol. Rep.* **2015**, *67*, 1090–1097. [CrossRef]
189. Tsai, M.-S.; Wang, Y.-H.; Lai, Y.-Y.; Tsou, H.-K.; Liou, G.-G.; Ko, J.-L.; Wang, S.-H. Kaempferol protects against propacetamol-induced acute liver injury through CYP2E1 inactivation, UGT1A1 activation, and attenuation of oxidative stress, inflammation and apoptosis in mice. *Toxicol. Lett.* **2018**, *290*, 97–109. [CrossRef]
190. Kluska, M.; Juszczak, M.; Wysokiński, D.; Żuchowski, J.; Stochmal, A.; Woźniak, K. Kaempferol derivatives isolated from Lens culinaris Medik. reduce DNA damage induced by etoposide in peripheral blood mononuclear cells. *Toxicol. Res.* **2019**, *8*, 896–907. [CrossRef]
191. Basu, A.; Das, A.S.; Sharma, M.; Pathak, M.P.; Chattopadhyay, P.; Biswas, K.; Mukhopadhyay, R. STAT3 and NF-κB are common targets for kaempferol-mediated attenuation of COX-2 expression in IL-6-induced macrophages and carrageenan-induced mouse paw edema. *Biochem. Biophys. Rep.* **2017**, *12*, 54–61. [CrossRef]
192. Ansó, E.; Zuazo, A.; Irigoyen, M.; Urdaci, M.C.; Rouzaut, A.; Martínez-Irujo, J.J. Flavonoids inhibit hypoxia-induced vascular endothelial growth factor expression by a HIF-1 independent mechanism. *Biochem. Pharmacol.* **2010**, *79*, 1600–1609. [CrossRef] [PubMed]
193. Seo, S.-H.; Jeong, G.-S. Fisetin inhibits TNF-α-induced inflammatory action and hydrogen peroxide-induced oxidative damage in human keratinocyte HaCaT cells through PI3K/AKT/Nrf-2-mediated heme oxygenase-1 expression. *Int. Immunopharmacol.* **2015**, *29*, 246–253. [CrossRef] [PubMed]
194. Althunibat, O.Y.; Al Hroob, A.M.; Abukhalil, M.H.; Germoush, M.O.; Bin-Jumah, M.; Mahmoud, A.M. Fisetin ameliorates oxidative stress, inflammation and apoptosis in diabetic cardiomyopathy. *Life Sci.* **2019**, *221*, 83–92. [CrossRef]
195. Hou, W.; Hu, S.; Su, Z.; Wang, Q.; Meng, G.; Guo, T.; Zhang, J.; Gao, P. Myricetin attenuates LPS-induced inflammation in RAW 264.7 macrophages and mouse models. *Future Med. Chem.* **2018**, *10*, 2253–2264. [CrossRef]

196. Zhang, M.-J.; Su, H.; Yan, J.-Y.; Li, N.; Song, Z.-Y.; Wang, H.-J.; Huo, L.-G.; Wang, F.; Ji, W.-S.; Qu, X.-J.; et al. Chemopreventive effect of Myricetin, a natural occurring compound, on colonic chronic inflammation and inflammation-driven tumorigenesis in mice. *Biomed. Pharmacother.* **2018**, *97*, 1131–1137. [CrossRef]
197. Chen, X.; Li, X.-F.; Chen, Y.; Zhu, S.; Li, H.-D.; Chen, S.-Y.; Wang, J.-N.; Pan, X.-Y.; Bu, F.-T.; Huang, C.; et al. Hesperetin derivative attenuates CCl4-induced hepatic fibrosis and inflammation by Gli-1-dependent mechanisms. *Int. Immunopharmacol.* **2019**, *76*, 105838. [CrossRef]
198. Samie, A.; Sedaghat, R.; Baluchnejadmojarad, T.; Roghani, M. Hesperetin, a citrus flavonoid, attenuates testicular damage in diabetic rats via inhibition of oxidative stress, inflammation, and apoptosis. *Life Sci.* **2018**, *210*, 132–139. [CrossRef]
199. Cheng, A.-W.; Tan, X.; Sun, J.-Y.; Gu, C.-M.; Liu, C.; Guo, X. Catechin attenuates TNF-α induced inflammatory response via AMPK-SIRT1 pathway in 3T3-L1 adipocytes. *PLoS ONE* **2019**, *14*, e0217090. [CrossRef]
200. Zhang, T.; Mu, Y.; Yang, M.; Al Maruf, A.; Li, P.; Li, C.; Dai, S.; Lu, J.; Dong, Q. (+)-Catechin prevents methylglyoxal-induced mitochondrial dysfunction and apoptosis in EA.hy926 cells. *Arch. Physiol. Biochem.* **2017**, *123*, 121–127. [CrossRef]
201. Knaze, V.; Zamora-Ros, R.; Luján-Barroso, L.; Romieu, I.; Scalbert, A.; Slimani, N.; Riboli, E.; Van Rossum, C.T.M.; Bueno-de-Mesquita, H.B.; Trichopoulou, A.; et al. Intake estimation of total and individual flavan-3-ols, proanthocyanidins and theaflavins, their food sources and determinants in the European Prospective Investigation into Cancer and Nutrition (EPIC) study. *Br. J. Nutr.* **2012**, *108*, 1095–1108. [CrossRef]
202. Márquez Campos, E.; Jakobs, L.; Simon, M.-C. Antidiabetic Effects of Flavan-3-ols and Their Microbial Metabolites. *Nutrients* **2020**, *12*, 1592. [CrossRef] [PubMed]
203. Thilakarathna, W.P.D.W.; Rupasinghe, H.P.V. Microbial metabolites of proanthocyanidins reduce chemical carcinogen-induced DNA damage in human lung epithelial and fetal hepatic cells in vitro. *Food Chem. Toxicol.* **2019**, *125*, 479–493. [CrossRef]
204. Lei, L.; Yang, Y.; He, H.; Chen, E.; Du, L.; Dong, J.; Yang, J. Flavan-3-ols consumption and cancer risk: A meta-analysis of epidemiologic studies. *Oncotarget* **2016**, *7*, 73573–73592. [CrossRef] [PubMed]
205. Gujar, K.; Wairkar, S. Nanocrystal technology for improving therapeutic efficacy of flavonoids. *Phytomedicine* **2020**, *71*, 153240. [CrossRef]
206. Cassidy, A.; Bertoia, M.; Chiuve, S.; Flint, A.; Forman, J.; Rimm, E.B. Habitual intake of anthocyanins and flavanones and risk of cardiovascular disease in men. *Am. J. Clin. Nutr.* **2016**, *104*, 587–594. [CrossRef] [PubMed]
207. Zhu, Y.; Huang, X.; Zhang, Y.; Wang, Y.; Liu, Y.; Sun, R.; Xia, M. Anthocyanin Supplementation Improves HDL-Associated Paraoxonase 1 Activity and Enhances Cholesterol Efflux Capacity in Subjects With Hypercholesterolemia. *J. Clin. Endocrinol. Metab.* **2014**, *99*, 561–569. [CrossRef] [PubMed]
208. Zhu, Y.; Ling, W.; Guo, H.; Song, F.; Ye, Q.; Zou, T.; Li, D.; Zhang, Y.; Li, G.; Xiao, Y.; et al. Anti-inflammatory effect of purified dietary anthocyanin in adults with hypercholesterolemia: A randomized controlled trial. *Nutr. Metab. Cardiovasc. Dis.* **2013**, *23*, 843–849. [CrossRef] [PubMed]
209. Barchitta, M.; Maugeri, A.; La Mastra, C.; Rosa, M.C.L.; Favara, G.; Lio, R.M.S.; Agodi, A. Dietary Antioxidant Intake and Human Papillomavirus Infection: Evidence from a Cross-Sectional Study in Italy. *Nutrients* **2020**, *12*, 1384. [CrossRef]
210. De Ferrars, R.M.; Czank, C.; Zhang, Q.; Botting, N.P.; Kroon, P.A.; Cassidy, A.; Kay, C.D. The pharmacokinetics of anthocyanins and their metabolites in humans: Pharmacokinetics of a (13)C-labelled anthocyanin. *Br. J. Pharmacol.* **2014**, *171*, 3268–3282. [CrossRef]
211. Sudhakaran, M.; Doseff, A.I. The Targeted Impact of Flavones on Obesity-Induced Inflammation and the Potential Synergistic Role in Cancer and the Gut Microbiota. *Molecules* **2020**, *25*, 2477. [CrossRef]
212. Zhong, Y.; Song, B.; Zheng, C.; Zhang, S.; Yan, Z.; Tang, Z.; Kong, X.; Duan, Y.; Li, F. Flavonoids from Mulberry Leaves Alleviate Lipid Dysmetabolism in High Fat Diet-Fed Mice: Involvement of Gut Microbiota. *Microorganisms* **2020**, *8*, 860. [CrossRef] [PubMed]
213. Kamalifard, M.; Abbasalizadeh, S.; Mirghafourvand, M.; Bastani, P.; Gholizadeh Shamasbi, S.; Khodaei, L.; Gholizadeh, G. The effect of *Seidlitzia rosmarinus* (*eshnan*) on the prevention of recurrent cystitis in women of reproductive age: A randomized, controlled, clinical trial. *Phytother. Res.* **2020**, *34*, 418–427. [CrossRef] [PubMed]

214. Pintova, S.; Dharmupari, S.; Moshier, E.; Zubizarreta, N.; Ang, C.; Holcombe, R.F. Genistein combined with FOLFOX or FOLFOX–Bevacizumab for the treatment of metastatic colorectal cancer: Phase I/II pilot study. *Cancer Chemother. Pharmacol.* **2019**, *84*, 591–598. [CrossRef] [PubMed]
215. Curtis, P.J.; Van der Velpen, V.; Berends, L.; Jennings, A.; Feelisch, M.; Umpleby, A.M.; Evans, M.; Fernandez, B.O.; Meiss, M.S.; Minnion, M.; et al. Blueberries improve biomarkers of cardiometabolic function in participants with metabolic syndrome—Results from a 6-month, double-blind, randomized controlled trial. *Am. J. Clin. Nutr.* **2019**, *109*, 1535–1545. [CrossRef] [PubMed]
216. Bakuradze, T.; Tausend, A.; Galan, J.; Groh, I.A.M.; Berry, D.; Tur, J.A.; Marko, D.; Richling, E. Antioxidative activity and health benefits of anthocyanin-rich fruit juice in healthy volunteers. *Free Radic. Res.* **2019**, *53*, 1045–1055. [CrossRef]
217. Munguia, L.; Rubio-Gayosso, I.; Ramirez-Sanchez, I.; Ortiz, A.; Hidalgo, I.; Gonzalez, C.; Meaney, E.; Villarreal, F.; Najera, N.; Ceballos, G. High Flavonoid Cocoa Supplement Ameliorates Plasma Oxidative Stress and Inflammation Levels While Improving Mobility and Quality of Life in Older Subjects: A Double-Blind Randomized Clinical Trial. *J. Gerontol. Ser. A* **2019**, *74*, 1620–1627. [CrossRef]
218. Zhang, H.; Gordon, R.; Li, W.; Yang, X.; Pattanayak, A.; Fowler, G.; Zhang, L.; Catalona, W.J.; Ding, Y.; Xu, L.; et al. Genistein treatment duration effects biomarkers of cell motility in human prostate. *PLoS ONE* **2019**, *14*, e0214078. [CrossRef]
219. Zhao, H.; Jia, L.; Chen, G.; Li, X.; Meng, X.; Zhao, X.; Xing, L.; Zhu, W. A prospective, three-arm, randomized trial of EGCG for preventing radiation-induced esophagitis in lung cancer patients receiving radiotherapy. *Radiother. Oncol.* **2019**, *137*, 186–191. [CrossRef]
220. Ud-Din, S.; Foden, P.; Mazhari, M.; Al-Habba, S.; Baguneid, M.; Bulfone-Paus, S.; McGeorge, D.; Bayat, A. A Double-Blind, Randomized Trial Shows the Role of Zonal Priming and Direct Topical Application of Epigallocatechin-3-Gallate in the Modulation of Cutaneous Scarring in Human Skin. *J. Investig. Dermatol.* **2019**, *139*, 1680–1690. [CrossRef]
221. Bazzucchi, I.; Patrizio, F.; Ceci, R.; Duranti, G.; Sgrò, P.; Sabatini, S.; Di Luigi, L.; Sacchetti, M.; Felici, F. The Effects of Quercetin Supplementation on Eccentric Exercise-Induced Muscle Damage. *Nutrients* **2019**, *11*, 205. [CrossRef]
222. Karbasforooshan, H.; Hosseini, S.; Elyasi, S.; Fani Pakdel, A.; Karimi, G. Topical silymarin administration for prevention of acute radiodermatitis in breast cancer patients: A randomized, double-blind, placebo-controlled clinical trial: Topical silymarin for prevention of radiodermatitis in breast cancer. *Phytother. Res.* **2019**, *33*, 379–386. [CrossRef] [PubMed]
223. Kim, S.B.; Pandita, R.K.; Eskiocak, U.; Ly, P.; Kaisani, A.; Kumar, R.; Cornelius, C.; Wright, W.E.; Pandita, T.K.; Shay, J.W. Targeting of Nrf2 induces DNA damage signaling and protects colonic epithelial cells from ionizing radiation. *Proc. Natl. Acad. Sci. USA* **2012**, *109*, E2949–E2955. [CrossRef] [PubMed]

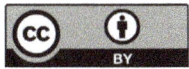

© 2020 by the authors. Licensee MDPI, Basel, Switzerland. This article is an open access article distributed under the terms and conditions of the Creative Commons Attribution (CC BY) license (http://creativecommons.org/licenses/by/4.0/).

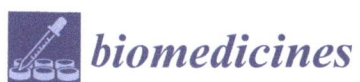

Article

Verbascoside Protects Pancreatic β-Cells against ER-Stress

Alessandra Galli [1,†], Paola Marciani [1,†], Algerta Marku [1], Silvia Ghislanzoni [1], Federico Bertuzzi [2], Raffaella Rossi [3], Alessia Di Giancamillo [3], Michela Castagna [1] and Carla Perego [1,*]

[1] Department of Pharmacological and Biomolecular Sciences, Università degli Studi di Milano, 20134 Milan, Italy; alessandra.galli1@unimi.it (A.G.); paola.marciani@unimi.it (P.M.); Algerta.marku@unimi.it (A.M.); silvia.ghislanzoni1@studenti.unimi.it (S.G.); michela.castagna@unimi.it (M.C.)
[2] Diabetology Unit, Niguarda Hospital, 20162 Milan, Italy; federico.bertuzzi@ospedaleniguarda.it
[3] Department of Veterinary Medicine, Università degli Studi di Milano, 26900 Lodi, Italy; raffaella.rossi@unimi.it (R.R.); alessia.digiancamillo@unimi.it (A.D.G.)
* Correspondence: Carla.Perego@unimi.it
† These authors contributed equally to this work.

Received: 16 November 2020; Accepted: 5 December 2020; Published: 8 December 2020

Abstract: Substantial epidemiological evidence indicates that a diet rich in polyphenols protects against developing type 2 diabetes. The phenylethanoid glycoside verbascoside/acteoside, a widespread polyphenolic plant compound, has several biological properties including strong antioxidant, anti-inflammatory and neuroprotective activities. The aim of this research was to test the possible effects of verbascoside on pancreatic β-cells, a target never tested before. Mouse and human β-cells were incubated with verbascoside (0.8–16 µM) for up to five days and a combination of biochemical and imaging techniques were used to assess the β-cell survival and function under normal or endoplasmic reticulum (ER)-stress inducing conditions. We found a dose-dependent protective effect of verbascoside against oxidative stress in clonal and human β-cells. Mechanistic studies revealed that the polyphenol protects β-cells against ER-stress mediated dysfunctions, modulating the activation of the protein kinase RNA-like endoplasmic reticulum kinase (PERK) branch of the unfolded protein response and promoting mitochondrial dynamics. As a result, increased viability, mitochondrial function and insulin content were detected in these cells. These studies provide the evidence that verbascoside boosts the ability of β-cells to cope with ER-stress, an important contributor of β-cell dysfunction and failure in diabetic conditions and support the therapeutic potential of verbascoside in diabetes.

Keywords: verbascoside; polyphenols; insulin-producing cells; diabetes; UPR; oxidative stress; ER-stress; PERK; anti-inflammatory; mitochondria

1. Introduction

Diabetes is a chronic disorder affecting hundreds of million people [1]. Different etiology characterizes Type 1 (T1D) and Type 2 diabetes (T2D) both featuring lack of insulin [2]. Insulin regulates plasma glucose concentration stimulating glucose uptake in muscle and fat cells and modulating liver glucose metabolism. Nutrient availability, hormones, and neural inputs regulate pancreatic insulin secretion and maintain blood glucose concentrations within a physiological range [3–5]. Therefore, β-cell dysfunction leads to diabetes characterized by fasting hyperglycemia.

T2D is a progressive condition in which insulin resistance and β-cells misfunctions are linked together and recent evidence rose interest in the critical primary role of β-cells to the hyperglycemic status [6,7]. In non-diabetic obese subjects β-cells compensate insulin resistance with increased secretion of the hormone. However, in some subjects, as their conditions deteriorate, insulinemia drops and glucose level climbs to hyperglycemia [8,9].

Glucose is the most important modulator of β-cell functions. Glucose stimulation affects regulation of genes and expression of proteins involved in many cell functions such as glycolysis, insulin synthesis and secretion [10]. Glucose-induced insulin secretion relies on oxidative metabolism to produce adenosine triphosphate (ATP) and a low level of reactive oxygen species (ROS) is physiologically produced. However, β-cells are not very well equipped with scavenger enzymes and this weakness makes them very susceptible to oxidative stress [11,12]. As oxidative stress climbs β-cells insulin production declines, and β-cells produce cytokines that ignite cell damage through inflammation and apoptosis [13]. Interestingly, although the reduced β-cells mass has been previously attributed to cell death, recent studies suggest a major role of cell dedifferentiation [14,15]. It has become clear that several stages drive to T2D. Metabolic and oxidative insults cause endoplasmic reticulum (ER) stress which leads to decline of insulin synthesis and secretion, inflammation processes follow the release of cytokines and β-cells loss may occur through apoptosis and dedifferentiation. This knowledge is fundamental in order to develop appropriate strategies of treatment, since oxidative stress and inflammation can be counteracted, and the plasticity of pancreatic cells allows the possibility to revert stem cells to β-cells as proved in mice [16].

Recently, the vulnerability of β-cells to oxidative stress has successfully prompted the use of dietary antioxidants to prevent diabetes [17]. Among the most interesting antioxidant food, olive oil is known for its beneficial properties since the ancient Greeks. Olive oil contains good amount of mono-unsaturated fatty acids (MUFA) and several polyphenols such as tyrosol, hydroxytyrosol, oleuropein, and verbascoside.

Verbascoside, also known as acteoside, is a phenylethanoid glycoside extracted from *Olea europea*, plants of the *Verbascum* species, and 23 other plant families [18–20]. It can also be obtained from olive oil by-products (it is enriched in olive-mill wastewater derived from olive fruit processing) or be produced by metabolic engineering and synthetic biology approaches [21].

No data have been reported about verbascoside bioavailability in humans, yet. Studies conducted on mice, SKBR3 and Caco-2 cells suggest that it may be feasible for non-metabolized verbascoside to cross the intestinal barrier, circulate in blood plasma, and exert antioxidant effects [20,22,23]. Unlike most of plant polyphenols, verbascoside mainly acts on cells through the modulation of gene transcription of a variety of enzymes and regulatory factors, with antioxidant and anti-inflammatory effects [24–30].

Although many beneficial effects of verbascoside for human health are known, there are no data about its effect on pancreatic β-cells. Since oxidative stress and inflammation are at the basis of T2D pathogenesis, we investigated whether verbascoside treatment might improve β-cells viability and function in ER-stress inducing conditions and we characterized the molecular mechanisms of its action. Our data reveal that verbascoside prevents β-cells oxidative stress and inflammation modulating the activation of the unfolded protein response and promoting mitochondrial dynamics, thus resulting in increased β-cell viability and insulin content.

2. Materials and Methods

2.1. Cells Culture and Materials

Mouse βtc3 cells (kindly provided by Prof. Hanahan—Department of Biochemistry and Biophysics, University of California, San Francisco, CA [31]) were cultured in RPMI 1640 medium (Euroclone S.p.A, ECB900, Pero MI, Italy) supplemented with 10% (v/v) heat-inactivated fetal calf serum (Euroclone S.p.A, ECS0180L, Pero MI, Italy), 1% (v/v) penicillin-streptomycin (EuroClone S.p.A., ECB3001D, Pero MI, Italy) and 1% (v/v) L-glutamine (EuroClone S.p.A., ECB300D, Pero MI, Italy). Human islets of Langerhans were isolated in Milan (Niguarda Ca' Granda) from cadaveric multiorgan donors according to the procedure described by Ricordi et al. [32]; they were cultured in RPMI culture medium containing

5.5 mmol/L glucose, 10% heat-inactivated fetal bovine serum, 0.7 mM Glutamine, 50 units/mL penicillin and 50 µg/mL streptomycin (EuroClone, S.p.A., Pero MI, Italy). Four different islets preparation were used, islets purity was 80 ± 10%. Islet isolation and islet studies were approved by the Ethics Committee of the Niguarda Ca' Granda hospital in Milan (11.12.2009).

βtc3 cells were treated with 0.8, 1.6, and 16 µM verbascoside (Carbosynth, OV08034, Compton, UK), caffeic acid and hydroxytyrosol (kind gift of Prof. Dell'Agli, Department of Pharmacological and Biomolecular Sciences, Università degli Studi di Milano, Milan, Italy) in complete RPMI medium for 5 days, while human islets with 16 µM verbascoside. Methanol/ethanol treated cells were used as controls. In order to induce oxidative stress, cells were treated with H_2O_2 (Sigma Aldrich, H1009, St. Louis MO, USA) 500 µM in complete RPMI medium for 20 min before analysis, while treatment with tunicamycin 2 µg/mL (T7765, Sigma Aldrich) for 7 h was performed to induce ER stress.

2.2. Detection of Cell Viability by MTT Test

Cells were plated in 96 multi-well plates, and five days after verbascoside treatment they were incubated with 0.5 mg/mL MTT (3-(4,5-dimethyltiazol-2-yl)-2,5-diphenyltetrazolium bromide) (Sigma-Aldrich, M5655, St. Louis, MO, USA) for 4 h in humidified atmosphere containing 5% of CO_2 at 37 °C. After incubation, cells were gently resuspended in 100 µL DMSO (Euro-Clone S.p.A., BK12611S, Pero MI, Italy) and the absorbance at 540 nm was detected with a microplate reader (Benchmark, microplate reader, Bio-Rad Laboratories, Hercules CA, USA) [33]. Experiments were performed in triplicate and data were expressed as fold increase over control samples.

2.3. Detection of Cell Death by Flow Cytometry

Five days after incubation with 16 µM verbascoside, the β-cells were detached by 7 min incubation with trypsin/EDTA, collected and centrifuged; the pellet was gently resuspended in phosphate buffer saline low salts. Cells were stained with Muse™ count and viability reagent (Millipore, MCH100102, Burlington MA, USA) following the manufacturer's protocol and analyzed through flow cytometry. Experiments were performed in triplicate and data were expressed as percentage of dead cells over the total.

2.4. ROS Generation

Intracellular ROS were evaluated with DCFDA (2′,7′-dichlorofuorescein diacetate) (Sigma Aldrich, D6883, St. Louis, MO, USA), a membrane permeable probe that becomes fluorescent when tied to ROS [34]. βtc3 cells were pre-loaded with 15 µM DCFDA in Krebs–Ringer buffer (125 mM NaCl, 5 mM KCl, 1.2 mM $MgSO_4$, 1.2 mM KH_2PO_4, 25 mM HEPES-NaOH pH 7.4 and 2 mM $CaCl_2$) supplemented with 11 mM glucose for 1 h at 37 °C. The ROS content was detected for 30 min both in basal and stress conditions with a microplate reader (485/528 nm Ex/Em) (TECAN Infinite® F500, Tecan Group Ltd. Männedorf, Switzerland). Mean values and standard deviations were based on three independent experiments.

2.5. Western Blotting

βtc3 cells were collected and solubilized in RIPA buffer (150 mM NaCl, 50 mM Tris HCl pH 7.6, 1 mM EDTA, 1% TERGITOL™ NP40, 0.5% deoxycholate) added with aprotinin (Sigma Aldrich, A4529, St. Louis, MO, USA), PMSF (Sigma Aldrich, 10837091001, St. Louis, MO, USA) and Roche inhibitors (Sigma Aldrich, 5892953001, St. Louis, MO, USA) for 40 min at 4 °C. Protein concentration was determined by Bradford assay [35] by using Bradford Reagent (Sigma Aldrich, B6916, St. Louis, MO, USA), 30 µg of proteins were resolved by 10% SDS-PAGE and transferred onto nitrocellulose membranes (Millipore, Burlington MA, USA). Primary antibodies were applied for 2 h in blocking buffer with 5% non-fat milk or 5% BSA solutions; the following primary antibodies were used: mouse anti-β-actin (Novus International Inc., NB600501, St. Louis, MO, USA), mouse anti-acrolein (Abcam, ab48501, Cambridge, UK), mouse anti-BIP (kind gift of Prof. Borgese Nica, Institute of Neuroscience, CNR,

Milan, Italy), rabbit anti-HNE (α-diagnostic International Inc., HNE11S, San Antonio, TX, USA), mouse anti-HSP70 (Enzo Life Sciences Inc., C92F3A-5, Farmingdale, NY, USA), rabbit anti-phospho-IκBα (Ser32) (Cell Signaling Technology Inc., 3033, Danvers, MA, USA), mouse anti-IκBα (Cell Signaling Technology Inc., 4814, Danvers, MA, USA), rabbit anti-phospho-NFκB p65 (Ser 536) (Cell Signaling Technology Inc., 3033, Danvers, MA, USA), rabbit anti-NFkB p65 (Cell Signaling Technology Inc., 8242, Danvers MA, USA), sheep anti-SOD1 (Merck, KGaA, Darmstadt, Germania), rabbit anti-PERK (Cell Signaling Technology Inc., 3192, Danvers, MA, USA), rabbit anti-eIF2α (Cell Signaling Technology Inc., 5324, Danvers, MA, USA) and rabbit anti-P-eIF2α (Ser 51) (Cell Signaling Technology Inc., 3597, Danvers, MA, USA). The secondary antibodies HRP-conjugated (Dako Agilent, Santa Clara, CA, USA) were used at 1:5000 dilution. Proteins were detected by using the ECL detection system (Euro-Clone S.p.A., Pero MI, Italy) by using Odyssey Fc Image system (LI-COR Biotechnology GmbH, Bad Homburg, Germany) and band density was quantified by Image Studio™ Lite software (LI-COR Biosciences, Lincoln, NE, USA) [36]. Experiments were performed in triplicate and data were expressed as fold increase over control samples.

2.6. Mitochondrial Membrane Potential

βtc3 cells and human islets of Langerhans were incubated with 100 nM MitoSpy™ Orange CMTMRos (BioLegend, 424803, Campoverde Srl, Milan, Italy) or 100 μM MitoSpy™ Green FM (BioLegend, 424805, Campoverde Srl, Milan, Italy) for 30 min at 37 °C; fluorescence intensities were detected with the microplate reader TECAN Infinite® F500 (551/576 nm Ex/Em for MitoSpy™ Orange CMTMRos; 490/516 nm Ex/Em for MitoSpy™ Green) (TECAN Infinite® F500, Tecan Group Ltd. Männedorf, Switzerland). Cells were incubated with 500 μM H_2O_2 for 20 min and fluorescence intensity was detected as previously described. Mean values and standard deviations were based on three different experiments.

2.7. Mitochondrial Morphology and Dynamics

βtc3 cells were pre-loaded with 100 nM MitoSpy™ Orange CMTMRos (BioLegend, 424803, Campoverde Srl, Milan, Italy) in 11 mM glucose Krebs–Ringer buffer at 37 °C for 30 min. Samples were positioned in an imaging chamber and random fields were imaged by using the rhodan filter of the Axio Observer Z1 microscope (Zeiss, Oberkochen Germany). To evaluate mitochondrial morphology, the following parameters were analyzed by using the ImageJ particle analyzer software: area (μm^2), circularity ($4\pi Area^2/Perimeter^2$) and Feret's maximum diameter (μm) [37].

For time-lapse experiments, single-cell imaging was carried out at 1 frame per second for 30 s under control or oxidative stress conditions. To measure the mitochondrial cumulative distance (μm^2), images were first corrected for photo bleaching, then videos were analyzed by using an existing Image-Pro Plus Plug-in (object tracking) (Media Cybernetics, Rockville, MD, USA). Up to twelve cells were imaged in three independent experiments and data were presented as mean values and standard deviations.

2.8. Insulin Secretion

Human isolated islets of Langerhans were seeded in 96-well plate at a density of 20 islets per well and, after 5 days of treatment, insulin content and secretion were measured in basal (3.3 mM glucose) and stimulated (16.7 mM glucose) conditions by means of an ELISA immunoassay (Mercodia, 10-1113-01, Uppsala, Sweden).

2.9. Statistical Analyses

All statistical analyses were performed with GraphPad Prism 8.0 on independent biological replicates. Means between two groups were evaluated by using the two-tailed Student's t-test and a p-value < 0.05 was taken as evidence of statistical significance. Means among three or more groups were compared by analysis of variance (ANOVA), followed by multiple post-hoc (Tukey's) comparison test. The statistical test used, exact P values and the number of replica (n) are indicated in the individual figure legends. Error bars in the figures display the mean ± S.D. or the mean ± S.E., as indicated.

3. Results

3.1. Verbascoside Improves β-Cells Viability

Since there were no data on verbascoside effect on β-cells, we performed MTT test to evaluate cell viability and as shown in Figure 1A, a positive dose-dependent trend was observed. Hence, for further studies, we selected the 16 μM concentration that statistically was proven effective to enhance β-cells viability.

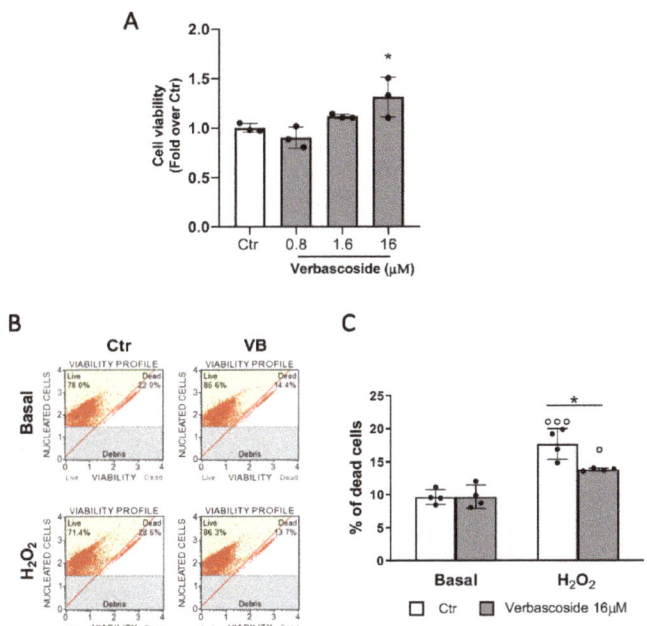

Figure 1. Verbascoside improves β-cell viability. Mouse βtc3 cells were treated with 0.8, 1.6, and 16 μM verbascoside (VB) for 5 days and methanol treated cells were used as controls. (**A**) MTT test. Data of three independent experiments (mean values ± SD) are expressed as fold change over control. (One-way ANOVA, post-hoc Tukey's test * $p = 0.046$ VB vs. Ctr). (**B**) Representative images of flow cytometry experiments. βtc3 cells were trypsinized, labelled with Muse^{TM} count and viability reagent, and analyzed through flow cytometry. Plot organization. Lower panel: cellular debris; upper panel: percentage of live (right part) and dead (left part) cells. (**C**) Quantification of β-cell death by flow cytometry. Data (mean values ± SD) are expressed as percentage of dead cells over total cells; experiments were performed in quadruplicate (two-way ANOVA, post-hoc Tukey's test. ° $p = 0.012$, °°° $p < 0.0001$ H_2O_2 vs. Basal; * $p = 0.018$ VB vs. Ctr).

By flow cytometry we studied the impact of five days incubation of verbascoside on β-cell survival in basal conditions and after 20 min of pre-treatment with 500 μM H_2O_2. In the basal condition, verbascoside did not affect cell survival, suggesting that the increased β-cell viability observed in the MTT assay may be due to improved mitochondrial activity. Whereas, after H_2O_2 exposure, 16 μM verbascoside pre-treatment significantly reduced oxidative stress-induced β-cell death (Figure 1B,C).

Verbascoside is a complex molecule that can be modified by hydrolyzing enzymes [18]. To test whether verbascoside metabolites could be responsible for the observed protective effect, βtc3 cells were treated with hydroxytyrosol and caffeic acids (0.8 and 16 µM) for 5 days. Both metabolites did not enhance cell viability, on the contrary a cytotoxic effect, more relevant after H_2O_2 exposure, was detected for the 16 µM concentration (Figure S1). This finding proves that verbascoside and not its metabolites exerts the protective effect to H_2O_2 treatment.

3.2. Verbascoside Modulates the Redox Homeostasis and Exerts an Anti-Inflammatory Effect in β-Cells

We first confirmed in βtc3 cells the anti-inflammatory and anti-oxidant effects of verbascoside observed in other cell types [24,29,34]. The verbascoside ROS scavenging activity was evaluated with βtc3 cells labelled with the ROS specific DCFDA (2′,7′-dichlorofuorescein diacetate) cellular permeable probe. As shown in Figure 2A, a significant decrease of ROS content was detected after verbascoside pre-treatment, both under basal and oxidative stress conditions.

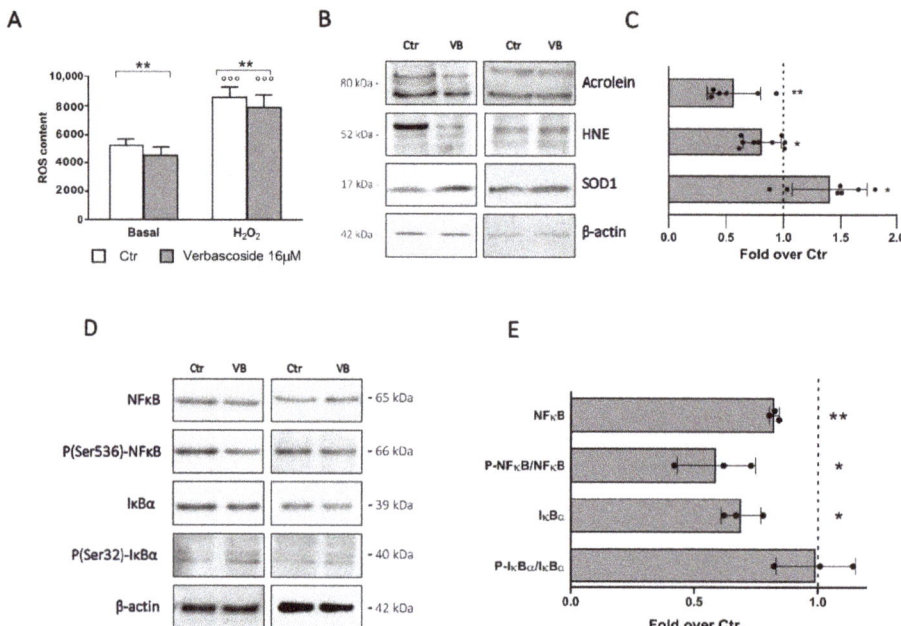

Figure 2. Verbascoside modulates redox homeostasis and inflammation in βtc3 cells. (**A**) ROS content. Intracellular ROS were monitored by DCFDA and quantified by fluorimetry (485/528 nm Ex/Em) under basal and oxidative stress (H_2O_2 500 µM for 30 min) conditions. Data are expressed as mean ± SD of three independent experiments. (Two-way ANOVA, post-hoc Tukey's test. °°° $p < 0.0001$ H_2O_2 vs. Basal; ** $p = 0.0055$ VB vs. Ctr). (**B**) Western blotting analysis of HNE, acrolein and SOD1 in cells treated with 16 µM verbascoside (VB) for 5 days (30 µg protein/sample). On the left, the molecular-weight size markers in kDa are reported. (**C**) Quantitative analysis of protein expression shows upregulation of SOD1 and reduction of HNE and acrolein in cells treated with 16 µM verbascoside. Data (mean values ± SD) are expressed as fold change over control (dashed line). (n = 6–9 independent experiments). (Student's t-test * $p < 0.05$, ** $p < 0.01$ VB vs. Ctr). (**D**) Western blotting analysis of NFκB pathways selected proteins in cells treated with 16 µM verbascoside (VB) for 5 days (30 µg protein/sample). On the right, the molecular-weight size markers in kDa are reported. (**E**) Quantitative analysis of protein expression shows that verbascoside treatment downregulates the activation of the NFκB pathway. Data (mean values ± SD) are expressed as fold change over control (dashed line). (n = 3 independent experiments performed in triplicate), (Student's t-test * $p < 0.05$, ** $p < 0.01$ VB vs. Ctr).

Western blot analyses revealed a significant decrease of oxidative stress markers acrolein and 4-hydroxynonenal (HNE) expression in verbascoside-treated cells. In addition, we found an increase of superoxide dismutase (SOD1) expression, suggesting that verbascoside exerts its antioxidant activity probably with two different mechanisms, directly as a ROS scavenger and indirectly by inducing the expression of antioxidant enzymes (Figure 2B,C).

The anti-inflammatory effect of verbascoside on β-cells was assessed by evaluating the activation of the NFκB pathway, the most important pro-inflammatory pathway in these cells [38]. By western blot analysis we found a reduced expression of inhibitor of nuclear factor kappa B (IκBα) and nuclear factor kappa-light-chain-enhancer (NFκB), and a significant decrease of NFκB phosphorylation in pre-treated cells, backing the hypothesis of the verbascoside effectiveness to reduce cellular inflammation (Figure 2D,E).

3.3. Verbascoside Modulates the Unfolded Protein Response of β-Cells

We then analyzed in depth the molecular mechanism by which verbascoside exerts antioxidant and anti-inflammatory roles, focusing on the endoplasmic reticulum which is emerging as a key sensor of metabolic and stress signals in β-cells. Under stress conditions, the organelle mounts a homeostatic response, known as the unfolded protein response (UPR), aimed at recovering the ER function; however, the excessive activation of this pathway results in apoptosis [39,40].

Markers of increased ER stress are the upregulation of chaperones proteins and activation of the UPR response. Western blotting analysis of cells treated with verbascoside revealed decreased levels of the two chaperonins heat shock protein 70 (HSP70) and binding immunoglobulin protein (BIP) (Figure 3A,B). Furthermore, a significant reduction of protein kinase RNA-like ER kinase (PERK) expression and decreased phosphorylation of its downstream effector, the eukaryotic translation initiation factor 2 (eIF2α), were detected.

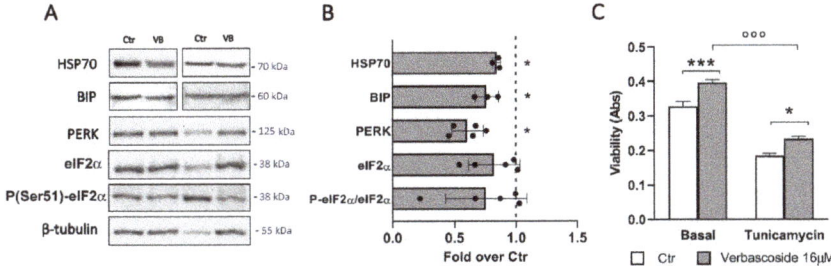

Figure 3. Verbascoside reduces ER stress. (**A**) Western blot analysis of ER stress markers in cells treated with 16 μM verbascoside (VB) for 5 days (30 μg protein/sample). On the right, the molecular-weight size markers in kDa are reported. (**B**) The quantitative analysis shows that verbascoside treatment reduces the expression of HSP70, BIP and PERK proteins. Data (mean values ± SD) are expressed as fold change over control (dashed line). (n = 3–5 independent experiments performed in triplicate) (Student's t-test * $p < 0.05$ vs. Ctr). (**C**) Mouse βtc3 cells were incubated with 16 μM verbascoside (VB) for 5 days and ER stress was induced by 2 μg/mL tunicamycin treatment for 7 h. MTT test reveals a protective role of verbascoside against the tunicamycin-induced ER stress. Data are expressed as mean ± SD of three independent experiments (two-way ANOVA, post-hoc Tukey's test. °°° $p < 0.0001$ tunicamycin vs. Basal; * $p = 0.024$ VB vs. Ctr; *** $p = 0.0001$).

Taken together, these data suggest that verbascoside protects β-cell from dysfunctions associated with ER-stress and acts by modulating the PERK branch of the UPR, a pathway deregulated in diabetes [41]. To confirm this hypothesis, the cells were treated with tunicamycin, an inhibitor of N-linked glycosylation and a potent ER-stress inducer (Figure 3C). As expected, a seven-hour incubation with 2 μg/mL tunicamycin increased the activation of the PERK pathway (Figure S2) and significantly reduced β-cell viability (Figure 3B). Interestingly, verbascoside pre-treatment (16 μM for

72 h) downregulated the expression of P-eIF2α and partially reverted the action of tunicamycin on β-cell viability.

Taken together these data strongly support a role of verbascoside in protecting β-cells by attenuation of ER-stress response.

3.4. Verbascoside Modulates β-Cells Mitochondrial Activity and Dynamics

MTT viability assays suggest a possible impact of verbascoside directly on mitochondria which ensure the coupling of insulin secretion to the nutritional state and the cell survival in this cell type. Shape and membrane potential are markers of the mitochondrial health [42]. We first evaluated mitochondrial membrane potential by labelling the cells with MitoSpy™ Orange CMTMRos, a permeable dye whose concentration depends on the inner mitochondrial membrane potential, while MitoSpy™ Green FM was used to normalize data to the mitochondrial mass (Figure 4A,B). Membrane potential of mitochondria in verbascoside-treated cells was increased compared to control in both basal and stress conditions. Interestingly, verbascoside metabolites exerted different effects. Caffeic acid did not improve the mitochondrial potential, whereas hydroxytyrosol caused a dose-dependent impairment of mitochondrial function, in agreement with data on cell viability, such an effect was more evident after H_2O_2 exposure (Figure S3).

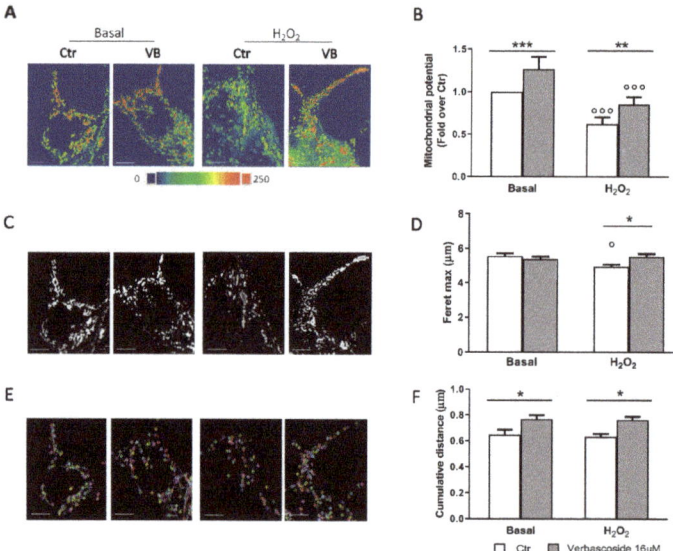

Figure 4. Verbascoside modulates mitochondrial activity, morphology and dynamics. Mouse βtc3 cells were treated with 16 μM verbascoside (VB) for 5 days and then loaded with 100 nM MitoSpy™ Orange CMTMRos. (**A**) Representative images of mitochondria in pseudocolors are shown (blue low intensity, red high intensity). Bar: 5 μm. (**B**) Quantitative analysis of mitochondrial membrane potential measured by fluorimetry (551/576 nm Ex/Em). Data (mean ± SD) were normalized to mitochondrial mass and expressed as fold change over control (n = 4 independent experiments). (Two-way ANOVA post-hoc Tukey's test °°° $p < 0.0001$ H_2O_2 vs. Basal; ** $p = 0.002$, *** $p = 0.0002$ VB vs. Ctr). (**C**) Representative epifluorescence images of mitochondria are shown. Bar: 5 μm. (**D**) Quantitative analysis of mitochondrial Feret's maximum diameter (μm); bars illustrate the average responses ± SEM (n = 10-15 cells in three independent experiments). (Two-way ANOVA, post-hoc Tukey's test. ° $p = 0.02$ H_2O_2 vs. Basal; * $p = 0.02$ VB vs. Ctr). (**E**) Video tracking of mitochondrial movements during the 30 s record. Bar: 5 μm. (**F**) Quantitative analyses of mitochondria movements. Bars illustrate the average response (cumulative distance) ± SEM of three independent experiments. (Two-way ANOVA, post-hoc Tukey's test. * $p = 0.02$ VB vs. Ctr).

Since function is strictly related to morphology, we measured the Feret's diameter, area, and circularity of the mitochondria. Acute oxidative stress promotes an extensive mitochondrial fission, thus resulting in smaller, circular mitochondria [42]. Under H_2O_2 stress condition, mitochondria of verbascoside-treated cells were more elongated and showed increased surface than control ones (Figure 4C,D and Figure S4). Mitochondrial circularity was lower in verbascoside-treated cells than in controls and differences were more evident in H_2O_2 treated cells (Figure S3), again confirming the protective role of the polyphenol.

The ability of these organelles to modify their shape in response to nutritional states or stressful conditions is under the control of fusion and fission events and requires mitochondrial motility [39]. Tracking of mitochondria movements led us to calculate the cumulative distance travelled and the analysis revealed a significant increase of mitochondria dynamics in the verbascoside treated cells when compared to control, already in basal conditions (Figure 4E,F and Videos S1–S4). The effect was more pronounced after H_2O_2 treatment, indeed verbascoside pre-treatment almost completely reverted the impact of oxidative stress on mitochondrial dynamics.

Taken together these data strongly support a key role of verbascoside in ensuring mitochondria dynamics which is crucial to promote the rapid adaptation of this organelle to stress conditions.

3.5. Verbascoside Impact on Human of Langerhans Survival and Function

Considering the translational potential of verbascoside application in human health, we verified its impact on human isolated islets of Langerhans, a more relevant model for physiopathological and pharmacological studies on β-cells. Isolated islets were treated with 16 μM verbascoside for 5 days and the mitochondrial membrane potential was evaluated. As reported in Figure 5A, while organelle potential was compromised in control human islets after H_2O_2 exposure, the inner membrane potential of mitochondria in verbascoside pre-treated islets did not decrease significantly, supporting the hypothesis of a protective role of verbascoside against ROS-induced β-cell dysfunction. Analysis of ER-stress markers expression showed an important reduction of P-eIF2α fraction in the two distinct islet preparations maintained in 16 μM verbascoside, confirming the downregulation of this pathway also in human samples (Figure 5D). The beneficial effects of the polyphenol treatment were corroborated by the increased insulin content observed in verbascoside-treated islets when compared to controls (Figure 5B). Data dispersion in our experiments did not allow to demonstrate any significant difference of glucose-stimulated insulin secretion (GSIS) in verbascoside-treated islets, although a positive trend seems apparent under both basal and stress conditions (Figure 5C).

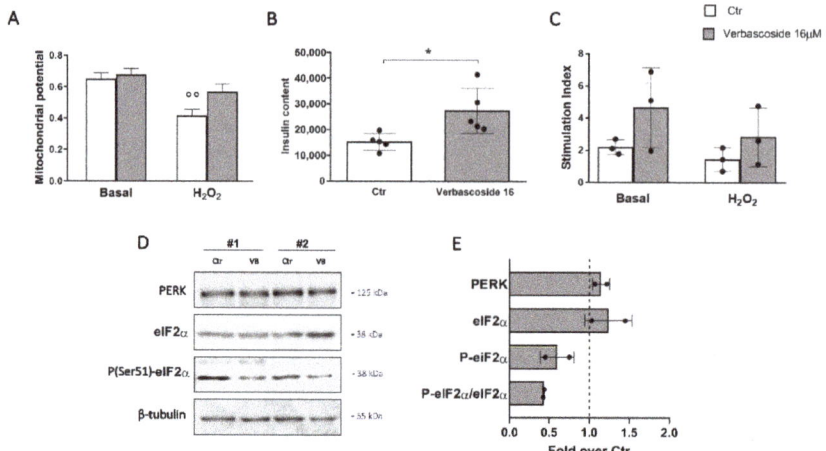

Figure 5. Verbascoside improves human islets of Langerhans function. Islets were incubated with or without 16 µM verbascoside for 5 days. (**A**) Mitochondrial membrane potential. Human islets were loaded with 100 nM MitoSpy™ Orange CMTMRos and 100 µM MitoSpy™ Green FM and the mitochondrial membrane potential and mass were measured by fluorimetry (551/576 nm Ex/Em and 490/516 nm Ex/Em, respectively). The bar graph illustrates the average responses ± SD, data were normalized to the mitochondrial mass (Two-way ANOVA, post-hoc Tukey's test, °° $p = 0.0013$ H_2O_2 vs. Basal). (**B**) The insulin content was evaluated by ELISA assay. Data (mean ± SD) are expressed as mU insulin/g protein (n = 5 independent experiments; Student's t-test, * $p < 0.05$ VB vs. Ctr). (**C**) The insulin release in basal (3.3 mM glucose) and stimulated (16.7 mM glucose) conditions were measured by ELISA assay and data (mean ± SD; n = 3 independent experiments) are expressed as stimulation index (stimulated/basal insulin release). (**D**) Western blot analysis of ER stress markers in islets treated with 16 µM verbascoside (VB) for 5 days (15 µg protein/sample). On the right, the molecular-weight size markers in kDa are reported. (**E**) The quantitative analysis shows a trend toward decrease of P-eIF2α expression and P-eIF2α/eIF2α ratio. Data (mean values ± SD) are expressed as fold change over control (dashed line). (n = 2 different islets isolation, performed in duplicate).

4. Discussion

Oxidative stress and inflammation are the basis of β-cell dysfunction occurring during T2D [43,44] as such, functional food, nutraceuticals, and phytochemicals have been investigated as tools to prevent type 2 diabetes [45]. In this work, we focused on verbascoside, that is known to exert anti-inflammatory and anti-oxidant activities in neurons [18]. Despite the high structural complexity, verbascoside and isoverbascoside have been found in blood plasma of rats fed with *Lippia citriodora* extract together with some metabolites [20]. In addition, cell accumulation of verbascoside and isoverbascoside has been detected in a breast cancer cell line SKBR3 [23] and studies conducted on Caco-2 cells demonstrate that moderate amounts of verbascoside and isoverbascoside remain intact and bioaccessible after in vitro digestive process. Furthermore, Caco-2 can uptake both molecules through a rapid and linear transport in 10 to 100 µM range [22]. No data have been reported about verbascoside bioavailability in humans, and yet the above-mentioned studies suggest that it may be feasible for non-metabolized verbascoside to cross intestinal barrier, circulate in blood plasma, and exert antioxidant effects on endocrine β-cells of the pancreas.

We found a dose-dependent (0.8–16 µM) protective role of verbascoside on clonal and human β-cells, both under basal and stress conditions. This effect is due to verbascoside itself and not to its metabolites caffeic acid and hydroxytyrosol, which actually appear cytotoxic at the 16 µM concentration. The concentrations proven active in our experiments are in line with those described in animals fed with verbascoside [20].

Though we do not know whether verbascoside acts extracellularly by binding to a membrane receptor or is internalized by endocytosis and works intracellularly, our data confirm that verbascoside has antioxidant and anti-inflammatory properties, and protects β-cells against ER-stress associated dysfunctions by reducing the UPR and promoting mitochondrial dynamics.

Indeed, we detected a significant decrease of ROS content in verbascoside treated cells which is further confirmed by the reduction of lipid peroxidation measured through HNE and acrolein expressions. Unlike most of plant polyphenols, verbascoside ROS scavenging activity mainly follows indirect (via upregulation of ROS removing enzymes) rather than direct pathways. In fact, it increases the gene transcription of some antioxidant enzymes through the activation of Nrf2 (NF-E2-related factor 2) pathway and via AhR (aryl hydrocarbon receptor)-dependent mechanism [24,29]. As such, we found increased expression of SOD1 in verbascoside treated cells.

ROS homeostasis is extremely relevant in β-cells pathology. Due to the shortage of antioxidant enzymes, elevated production of ROS cannot be neutralized and ER stress promoting protein misfolding is induced. ER stress leads to a reduction of insulin transcription and translation through the activation of the UPR [44,46]. This pathway has the main purpose of recovering the ER function through the reprogramming of gene expression, however when overstimulated, it triggers apoptosis. Our data suggest that an important action of verbascoside is to mitigate the UPR, allowing the modifications necessary to repair ER dysfunction, without causing apoptosis. According to this possibility, the expression of BIP, HSP70 and PERK proteins was decreased in verbascoside treated β-cells, and the activation of PERK pathway was attenuated in response to tunicamycin-induced ER stress. A similar action was reported for tyrosol in the insulinoma NIT-1 cell line [47].

Particularly interesting is the ability of verbascoside to modulate the activation of the PERK branch of the UPR. In β-cells this pathway is required to maintain the basal secretory homeostasis and β-cell survival, and it is severely deregulated in diabetes [41,48]. Even more intriguing, common variants at PERK contribute to the risk of prediabetes and recessive mutations in the EIF2AK3 gene (encoding PERK) underlie susceptibility to the Wolcott–Rallison syndrome characterized by permanent neonatal insulin dependent diabetes [49,50].

Downregulation of the IκBα-NFκB inflammatory pathway was also detected in our system in the presence of verbascoside. NFκB represents the main inflammatory pathway in β-cells and its sustained activation initiates a cascade of events culminating in β-cell death. In stressed β-cells, the reduction of NFκB expression protects pancreatic β-cells from diabetogenic agents [27,51], further supporting the verbascoside application in diabetes prevention. Interestingly, PERK signaling activates the transcription factors NFR2 (implicated in the redox homeostasis) and NFκB, thus explaining the anti-oxidant and anti-inflammatory effects of verbascoside [40,52].

Our data also reveal an important role of verbascoside on mitochondrial activity and dynamics. Marker of mitochondrial operational quality is their dynamic, a process characterized by coordinated cycles of fusion and fission events that regulates mitochondrial number, distribution, morphology and their membrane potential [39]. In line with this possibility, verbascoside improves βtc3 mitochondrial membrane potential both under basal and stress conditions. Again, the effect is due to verbascoside and not to its metabolites, as caffeic acid does not improve mitochondrial function and hydroxytyrosol significantly decreases the organelle potential. Increased mitochondrial dynamics and changes in their morphology were observed by tracking mitochondrial movements, thus suggesting that verbascoside promotes a mito-morphosis program. Reshaping of the cellular mitochondrial network affects the assembly of the respiratory chain super-complexes, thus altering not only the cell metabolism but also its redox state and enabling cells to better counteract oxidative stress and inflammation [5,37,39].

Although the molecular mechanism is still unknown, we can hypothesize that verbascoside, as other polyphenols, protects mitochondrial DNA by reducing ROS concentration [53] and prevents the opening of mitochondrial permeability transition pore [54], ensuring the physiological mitochondrial activity. Another intriguing possibility is that modification of mitochondria dynamics and activity is again mediated by the action of verbascoside on the UPR. Indeed, a recent research in the mitochondrial field indicates that sites of ER-mitochondria interaction play a key role in the control of mitochondrial dynamics and activity in response to oxidative stress and PERK is involved in the phenomenon [55].

Most in vitro studies with polyphenols were performed in cell lines, often of tumoral origin, which differ from original cells in terms of metabolism and ROS production. We here provide evidence that verbascoside exerts a protective effect also on human isolated islets of Langerhans, the final target of intervention in diabetes. Interestingly, the polyphenol mitigates the PERK signaling activation already under basal conditions, thus increasing the insulin content and preventing oxidative stress-mediated mitochondrial dysfunctions. It remains to be elucidated whether the polyphenol effect on insulin content reflects the compound ability to prevent β-cell death, to mitigate ER stress or to directly control the insulin gene expression, as shown for other polyphenolic compounds [56]. These data are particularly relevant considering the possible use of verbascoside as a complementary therapy in diabetes treatment.

5. Conclusions

The in vitro studies reported here on clonal and human β-cells, indicate that verbascoside exerts protective effects against ER-stress associated dysfunctions, mitigating the activation of the PERK branch of the UPR and improving mitochondria dynamics. As disruption of ER homeostasis triggers β-cells damage and diabetes, these data provide a rationale for the possible use of verbascoside as nutraceutical in disease prevention and treatment. Yet, many issues need to be resolved for an effective clinical application of verbascoside. Despite the wealth of laboratory studies, reliable clinical studies confirming the health effects of verbascoside in vivo are limited. Furthermore, increasing its stability and bioavailability is mandatory for the future application of this compound in human health. From this point, verbascoside is an interesting molecule because its scaffold has different reactive sites that can be modified by combinatory chemistry. We expect that the information resulting from these studies will open avenues for therapeutic modulation of oxidative stress and inflammation in pathological condition by using natural compounds.

Supplementary Materials: The following are available online at http://www.mdpi.com/2227-9059/8/12/582/s1. Figure S1: Effects of caffeic acid and hydroxytyrosol on β-cell viability. Figure S2: Effects of verbascoside on tunicamycin-induced ER stress. Figure S3: Effects of caffeic acid and hydroxytyrosol on mitochondrial membrane potential. Figure S4: Quantitative image analyses of mitochondria in cells treated with caffeic acid and hydroxytyrosol. Video S1,S2 Videos: Mitochondria dynamics recorded under basal conditions, in the absence (S1) or presence (S2) of verbascoside. Video S3, S4: Mitochondria dynamics recorded under oxidative stress conditions, in the absence (S3) or presence (S4) of verbascoside.

Author Contributions: Conceptualization, A.G., P.M. and C.P.; data curation, A.G. and P.M.; formal analysis, A.G. and P.M.; funding acquisition, C.P.; investigation, M.C.; methodology, A.M. and S.G.; resources, F.B., R.R. and A.D.G.; supervision, C.P.; validation, A.M., S.G. and M.C.; visualization, A.G. and A.M.; writing—original draft, A.G.; writing—review and editing, P.M., A.M., F.B., R.R., A.D.G., M.C. and C.P. All authors have read and agreed to the published version of the manuscript.

Funding: This research received no external funding.

Acknowledgments: We would like to thank Carlo Corino and Mario Dell'Agli for reagents and helpful discussion.

Conflicts of Interest: The authors declare no conflict of interest.

References

1. Cho, N.H.; Shaw, J.E.; Karuranga, S.; Huang, Y.; da Rocha Fernandes, J.D.; Ohlrogge, A.W.; Malanda, B. IDF Diabetes Atlas: Global estimates of diabetes prevalence for 2017 and projections for 2045. *Diabetes Res. Clin. Pract.* **2018**, *138*, 271–281. [CrossRef]
2. Leslie, R.D.; Palmer, J.; Schloot, N.C.; Lernmark, A. Diabetes at the crossroads: Relevance of disease classification to pathophysiology and treatment. *Diabetologia* **2016**, *59*, 13–20. [CrossRef] [PubMed]
3. Tokarz, V.L.; MacDonald, P.E.; Klip, A. The cell biology of systemic insulin function. *J. Cell Biol.* **2018**, *217*, 2273–2289. [CrossRef] [PubMed]

4. Perego, C.; Da Dalt, L.; Pirillo, A.; Galli, A.; Catapano, A.L.; Norata, G.D. Cholesterol metabolism, pancreatic β-cell function and diabetes. *Biochim. et Biophys. Acta (BBA) Mol. Basis Dis.* **2019**, *1865*, 2149–2156. [CrossRef] [PubMed]
5. Galli, A.; Algerta, M.; Marciani, P.; Schulte, C.; Lenardi, C.; Milani, P.; Maffioli, E.; Tedeschi, G.; Perego, C. Shaping Pancreatic β-Cell Differentiation and Functioning: The Influence of Mechanotransduction. *Cells* **2020**, *9*, 413. [CrossRef]
6. Ashcroft, F.M.; Rorsman, P. Diabetes Mellitus and the β Cell: The Last Ten Years. *Cell* **2012**, *148*, 1160–1171. [CrossRef] [PubMed]
7. Rosengren, A.H.; Braun, M.; Mahdi, T.; Andersson, S.A.; Travers, M.E.; Shigeto, M.; Zhang, E.; Almgren, P.; Ladenvall, C.; Axelsson, A.S.; et al. Reduced Insulin Exocytosis in Human Pancreatic -Cells With Gene Variants Linked to Type 2 Diabetes. *Diabetes* **2012**, *61*, 1726–1733. [CrossRef] [PubMed]
8. Polonsky, K.S. Dynamics of insulin secretion in obesity and diabetes. *Int. J. Obes.* **2000**, *24*, S29–S31. [CrossRef]
9. Roden, M.; Shulman, G.I. The integrative biology of type 2 diabetes. *Nature* **2019**, *576*, 51–60. [CrossRef]
10. Schrimpe-Rutledge, A.C.; Fontès, G.; Gritsenko, M.A.; Norbeck, A.D.; Anderson, D.J.; Waters, K.M.; Adkins, J.N.; Smith, R.D.; Poitout, V.; Metz, T.O. Discovery of novel glucose-regulated proteins in isolated human pancreatic islets using LC-MS/MS-based proteomics. *J. Proteome Res.* **2012**, *11*, 3520–3532. [CrossRef]
11. Gerber, P.A.; Rutter, G.A. The Role of Oxidative Stress and Hypoxia in Pancreatic Beta-Cell Dysfunction in Diabetes Mellitus. *Antioxid. Redox Signal.* **2017**, *26*, 501–518. [CrossRef] [PubMed]
12. Lenzen, S.; Drinkgern, J.; Tiedge, M. Low antioxidant enzyme gene expression in pancreatic islets compared with various other mouse tissues. *Free Radic. Biol. Med.* **1996**, *20*, 463–466. [CrossRef]
13. Butler, A.E.; Janson, J.; Bonner-Weir, S.; Ritzel, R.; Rizza, R.A.; Butler, P.C. Beta-cell deficit and increased beta-cell apoptosis in humans with type 2 diabetes. *Diabetes* **2003**, *52*, 102–110. [CrossRef] [PubMed]
14. Cinti, F.; Bouchi, R.; Kim-Muller, J.Y.; Ohmura, Y.; Sandoval, P.R.; Masini, M.; Marselli, L.; Suleiman, M.; Ratner, L.E.; Marchetti, P.; et al. Evidence of β-Cell Dedifferentiation in Human Type 2 Diabetes. *J. Clin. Endocrinol. Metab.* **2016**, *101*, 1044–1054. [CrossRef] [PubMed]
15. Dorrell, C.; Schug, J.; Canaday, P.S.; Russ, H.A.; Tarlow, B.D.; Grompe, M.T.; Horton, T.; Hebrok, M.; Streeter, P.R.; Kaestner, K.H.; et al. Human islets contain four distinct subtypes of β cells. *Nat. Commun.* **2016**, *7*, 11756. [CrossRef]
16. Wang, Z.; York, N.W.; Nichols, C.G.; Remedi, M.S. Pancreatic β cell dedifferentiation in diabetes and redifferentiation following insulin therapy. *Cell Metab.* **2014**, *19*, 872–882. [CrossRef]
17. Montonen, J.; Knekt, P.; Järvinen, R.; Reunanen, A. Dietary antioxidant intake and risk of type 2 diabetes. *Diabetes Care* **2004**, *27*, 362–366. [CrossRef]
18. Alipieva, K.; Korkina, L.; Orhan, I.E.; Georgiev, M.I. Verbascoside—A review of its occurrence, (bio)synthesis and pharmacological significance. *Biotechnol. Adv.* **2014**, *32*, 1065–1076. [CrossRef]
19. Alipieva, K.I.; Orhan, I.E.; Cankaya, I.I.T.; Kostadinova, E.P.; Georgiev, M.I. Treasure from garden: Chemical profiling, pharmacology and biotechnology of mulleins. *Phytochem. Rev.* **2014**, *13*, 417–444. [CrossRef]
20. Quirantes-Piné, R.; Herranz-López, M.; Funes, L.; Borrás-Linares, I.; Micol, V.; Segura-Carretero, A.; Fernández-Gutiérrez, A. Phenylpropanoids and their metabolites are the major compounds responsible for blood-cell protection against oxidative stress after administration of Lippia citriodora in rats. *Phytomedicine* **2013**, *20*, 1112–1118. [CrossRef]
21. Zhou, Y.; Zhu, J.; Shao, L.; Guo, M. Current advances in acteoside biosynthesis pathway elucidation and biosynthesis. *Fitoterapia* **2020**, *142*, 104495. [CrossRef] [PubMed]
22. Cardinali, A.; Linsalata, V.; Lattanzio, V.; Ferruzzi, M.G. Verbascosides from Olive Mill Waste Water: Assessment of Their Bioaccessibility and Intestinal Uptake Using an In Vitro Digestion/Caco-2 Model System. *J. Food Sci.* **2011**, *76*, H48–H54. [CrossRef] [PubMed]
23. Quirantes-Piné, R.; Zurek, G.; Barrajón-Catalán, E.; Bäßmann, C.; Micol, V.; Segura-Carretero, A.; Fernández-Gutiérrez, A. A metabolite-profiling approach to assess the uptake and metabolism of phenolic compounds from olive leaves in SKBR3 cells by HPLC-ESI-QTOF-MS. *J. Pharm. Biomed. Anal.* **2013**, *72*, 121–126. [CrossRef]
24. Korkina, L.; Kostyuk, V.; De Luca, C.; Pastore, S. Plant phenylpropanoids as emerging anti-inflammatory agents. *Mini Rev. Med. Chem.* **2011**, *11*, 823–835. [CrossRef]

25. Lee, J.H.; Lee, J.Y.; Kang, H.S.; Jeong, C.H.; Moon, H.; Whang, W.K.; Kim, C.J.; Sim, S.S. The effect of acteoside on histamine release and arachidonic acid release in RBL-2H3 mast cells. *Arch. Pharm. Res.* **2006**, *29*, 508–513. [CrossRef]
26. Lee, J.Y.; Woo, E.-R.; Kang, K.W. Inhibition of lipopolysaccharide-inducible nitric oxide synthase expression by acteoside through blocking of AP-1 activation. *J. Ethnopharmacol.* **2005**, *97*, 561–566. [CrossRef] [PubMed]
27. Mazzon, E.; Esposito, E.; Di Paola, R.; Riccardi, L.; Caminiti, R.; Dal Toso, R.; Pressi, G.; Cuzzocrea, S. Effects of verbascoside biotechnologically produced by Syringa vulgaris plant cell cultures in a rodent model of colitis. *Naunyn. Schmiedebergs Arch. Pharmacol.* **2009**, *380*, 79–94. [CrossRef] [PubMed]
28. Pastore, S.; Lulli, D.; Fidanza, P.; Potapovich, A.I.; Kostyuk, V.A.; De Luca, C.; Mikhal'chik, E.; Korkina, L.G. Plant polyphenols regulate chemokine expression and tissue repair in human keratinocytes through interaction with cytoplasmic and nuclear components of epidermal growth factor receptor system. *Antioxid. Redox Signal.* **2012**, *16*, 314–328. [CrossRef]
29. Potapovich, A.I.; Lulli, D.; Fidanza, P.; Kostyuk, V.A.; De Luca, C.; Pastore, S.; Korkina, L.G. Plant polyphenols differentially modulate inflammatory responses of human keratinocytes by interfering with activation of transcription factors NFκB and AhR and EGFR-ERK pathway. *Toxicol. Appl. Pharmacol.* **2011**, *255*, 138–149. [CrossRef]
30. Song, H.S.; Choi, M.Y.; Ko, M.S.; Jeong, J.M.; Kim, Y.H.; Jang, B.H.; Sung, J.H.; Kim, M.G.; Whang, W.K.; Sim, S.S. Competitive inhibition of cytosolic Ca2+-dependent phospholipase A2 by acteoside in RBL-2H3 cells. *Arch. Pharm. Res.* **2012**, *35*, 905–910. [CrossRef]
31. Di Cairano, E.S.; Davalli, A.M.; Perego, L.; Sala, S.; Sacchi, V.F.; La Rosa, S.; Finzi, G.; Placidi, C.; Capella, C.; Conti, P.; et al. The Glial Glutamate Transporter 1 (GLT1) Is Expressed by Pancreatic β-Cells and Prevents Glutamate-induced β-Cell Death. *J. Biol. Chem.* **2011**, *286*, 14007–14018. [CrossRef] [PubMed]
32. Ricordi, C.; Lacy, P.E.; Finke, E.H.; Olack, B.J.; Scharp, D.W. Automated method for isolation of human pancreatic islets. *Diabetes* **1988**, *37*, 413–420. [CrossRef]
33. Mosmann, T. Rapid colorimetric assay for cellular growth and survival: Application to proliferation and cytotoxicity assays. *J. Immunol. Methods* **1983**, *65*, 55–63. [CrossRef]
34. Cumaoğlu, A.; Rackova, L.; Stefek, M.; Kartal, M.; Maechler, P.; Karasu, C. Effects of olive leaf polyphenols against H_2O_2 toxicity in insulin secreting β-cells. *Acta Biochim. Pol.* **2011**, *58*, 45–50. [CrossRef] [PubMed]
35. Bradford, M.M. A rapid and sensitive method for the quantitation of microgram quantities of protein utilizing the principle of protein-dye binding. *Anal. Biochem.* **1976**, *72*, 248–254. [CrossRef]
36. Galli, A.; Maffioli, E.; Sogne, E.; Moretti, S.; Di Cairano, E.S.; Negri, A.; Nonnis, S.; Norata, G.D.; Bonacina, F.; Borghi, F.; et al. Cluster-assembled zirconia substrates promote long-term differentiation and functioning of human islets of Langerhans. *Sci. Rep.* **2018**, *8*, 9979. [CrossRef]
37. Maffioli, E.; Galli, A.; Nonnis, S.; Marku, A.; Negri, A.; Piazzoni, C.; Milani, P.; Lenardi, C.; Perego, C.; Tedeschi, G. Proteomic analysis reveals a mitochondrial remodeling of βTC3 cells in response to nanotopography. *Front. Cell Dev. Biol.* **2020**, *8*, 508. [CrossRef]
38. Melloul, D. Role of NF-κB in β-cell death. *Biochem. Soc. Trans.* **2008**, *36*, 334–339. [CrossRef] [PubMed]
39. Tilokani, L.; Nagashima, S.; Paupe, V.; Prudent, J. Mitochondrial dynamics: Overview of molecular mechanisms. *Essays Biochem.* **2018**, *62*, 341–360. [CrossRef] [PubMed]
40. Hotamisligil, G.S. Endoplasmic Reticulum Stress and the Inflammatory Basis of Metabolic Disease. *Cell* **2010**, *140*, 900–917. [CrossRef]
41. Cnop, M.; Toivonen, S.; Igoillo-Esteve, M.; Salpea, P. Endoplasmic reticulum stress and eIF2α phosphorylation: The Achilles heel of pancreatic β cells. *Mol. Metab.* **2017**, *6*, 1024–1039. [CrossRef] [PubMed]
42. Campello, S.; Scorrano, L. Mitochondrial shape changes: Orchestrating cell pathophysiology. *EMBO Rep.* **2010**, *11*, 678–684. [CrossRef]
43. Gothai, S.; Ganesan, P.; Park, S.-Y.; Fakurazi, S.; Choi, D.-K.; Arulselvan, P. Natural Phyto-Bioactive Compounds for the Treatment of Type 2 Diabetes: Inflammation as a Target. *Nutrients* **2016**, *8*, 461. [CrossRef] [PubMed]
44. Leibowitz, G.; Kaiser, N.; Cerasi, E. β-Cell failure in type 2 diabetes. *J. Diabetes Investig.* **2011**, *2*, 82–91. [CrossRef]
45. Martel, J.; Ojcius, D.M.; Chang, C.-J.; Lin, C.-S.; Lu, C.-C.; Ko, Y.-F.; Tseng, S.-F.; Lai, H.-C.; Young, J.D. Anti-obesogenic and antidiabetic effects of plants and mushrooms. *Nat. Rev. Endocrinol.* **2017**, *13*, 149–160. [CrossRef]

46. Hasnain, S.Z.; Prins, J.B.; McGuckin, M.A. Oxidative and endoplasmic reticulum stress in β-cell dysfunction in diabetes. *J. Mol. Endocrinol.* **2016**, *56*, R33–R54. [CrossRef]
47. Lee, H.; Im, S.W.; Jung, C.H.; Jang, Y.J.; Ha, T.Y.; Ahn, J. Tyrosol, an olive oil polyphenol, inhibits ER stress-induced apoptosis in pancreatic β-cell through JNK signaling. *Biochem. Biophysical. Res. Commun.* **2016**, *469*, 748–752. [CrossRef]
48. Gao, Y.; Sartori, D.J.; Li, C.; Yu, Q.-C.; Kushner, J.A.; Simon, M.C.; Diehl, J.A. PERK is required in the adult pancreas and is essential for maintenance of glucose homeostasis. *Mol. Cell Biol.* **2012**, *32*, 5129–5139. [CrossRef]
49. Delépine, M.; Nicolino, M.; Barrett, T.; Golamaully, M.; Mark Lathrop, G.; Julier, C. EIF2AK3, encoding translation initiation factor 2-α kinase 3, is mutated in patients with Wolcott-Rallison syndrome. *Nat. Genet.* **2000**, *25*, 406–409. [CrossRef]
50. Feng, N.; Ma, X.; Wei, X.; Zhang, J.; Dong, A.; Jin, M.; Zhang, H.; Guo, X. Common variants in PERK, JNK, BIP and XBP1 genes are associated with the risk of prediabetes or diabetes-related phenotypes in a Chinese population. *Chin. Med. J. (Engl.)* **2014**, *127*, 2438–2444.
51. Eldor, R.; Yeffet, A.; Baum, K.; Doviner, V.; Amar, D.; Ben-Neriah, Y.; Christofori, G.; Peled, A.; Carel, J.C.; Boitard, C.; et al. Conditional and specific NF- B blockade protects pancreatic beta cells from diabetogenic agents. *Proc. Natl. Acad. Sci. USA* **2006**, *103*, 5072–5077. [CrossRef] [PubMed]
52. Deng, J.; Lu, P.D.; Zhang, Y.; Scheuner, D.; Kaufman, R.J.; Sonenberg, N.; Harding, H.P.; Ron, D. Translational repression mediates activation of nuclear factor kappa B by phosphorylated translation initiation factor 2. *Mol. Cell Biol.* **2004**, *24*, 10161–10168. [CrossRef] [PubMed]
53. Fernández del Río, L.; Gutiérrez-Casado, E.; Varela-López, A.; Villalba, J.M. Olive Oil and the Hallmarks of Aging. *Molecules* **2016**, *21*, 163. [CrossRef]
54. Sandoval-Acuña, C.; Ferreira, J.; Speisky, H. Polyphenols and mitochondria: An update on their increasingly emerging ROS-scavenging independent actions. *Arch. Biochem. Biophys.* **2014**, *559*, 75–90. [CrossRef] [PubMed]
55. Verfaillie, T.; Rubio, N.; Garg, A.D.; Bultynck, G.; Rizzuto, R.; Decuypere, J.-P.; Piette, J.; Linehan, C.; Gupta, S.; Samali, A.; et al. PERK is required at the ER-mitochondrial contact sites to convey apoptosis after ROS-based ER stress. *Cell. Death Differ.* **2012**, *19*, 1880–1891. [CrossRef]
56. Kang, G.G.; Francis, N.; Hill, R.; Waters, D.; Blanchard, C.; Santhakumar, A.B. Dietary Polyphenols and Gene Expression in Molecular Pathways Associated with Type 2 Diabetes Mellitus: A Review. *Int. J. Mol. Sci.* **2019**, *21*, 140. [CrossRef]

Publisher's Note: MDPI stays neutral with regard to jurisdictional claims in published maps and institutional affiliations.

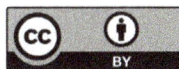

© 2020 by the authors. Licensee MDPI, Basel, Switzerland. This article is an open access article distributed under the terms and conditions of the Creative Commons Attribution (CC BY) license (http://creativecommons.org/licenses/by/4.0/).

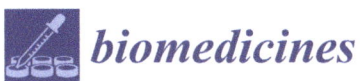

Review
Antiviral Effects of Polyphenols from Marine Algae

Natalya N. Besednova [1,*], Boris G. Andryukov [1,2], Tatyana S. Zaporozhets [1], Sergey P. Kryzhanovsky [3], Ludmila N. Fedyanina [2], Tatyana A. Kuznetsova [1], Tatyana N. Zvyagintseva [4] and Mikhail Yu. Shchelkanov [1,2,5,6]

[1] G.P. Somov Institute of Epidemiology and Microbiology, Russian Federal Service for Surveillance on Consumer Rights Protection and Human Wellbeing, 690087 Vladivostok, Russia; andrukov_bg@mail.ru (B.G.A.); niiem_vl@mail.ru (T.S.Z.); takuznets@mail.ru (T.A.K.); adorob@mail.ru (M.Y.S.)
[2] School of Biomedicine, Far Eastern Federal University (FEFU), 690091 Vladivostok, Russia; fedyanina.ln@dvfu.ru
[3] Medical Association of the Far Eastern Branch of the Russian Academy of Sciences, 690022 Vladivostok, Russia; priemmodvoran@mail.ru
[4] Elyakov Pacific Institute of Bioorganic Chemistry, FEB RAS, 690022 Vladivostok, Russia; zvyag@piboc.dvo.ru
[5] Federal Scientific Center of the Eastern Asia Terrestrial Biodiversity, Far Eastern Branch of Russian Academy of Sciences, 690091 Vladivostok, Russia
[6] National Scientific Center of Marine Biology, Far Eastern Branch of Russian Academy of Sciences, 690091 Vladivostok, Russia
* Correspondence: besednoff_lev@mail.ru; Tel.: +7-4232-442-446

Abstract: The disease-preventive and medicinal properties of plant polyphenolic compounds have long been known. As active ingredients, they are used to prevent and treat many noncommunicable diseases. In recent decades, marine macroalgae have attracted the attention of biotechnologists and pharmacologists as a promising and almost inexhaustible source of polyphenols. This heterogeneous group of compounds contains many biopolymers with unique structure and biological properties that exhibit high anti-infective activity. In the present review, the authors focus on the antiviral potential of polyphenolic compounds (phlorotannins) from marine algae and consider the mechanisms of their action as well as other biological properties of these compounds that have effects on the progress and outcome of viral infections. Effective nutraceuticals, to be potentially developed on the basis of algal polyphenols, can also be used in the complex therapy of viral diseases. It is necessary to extend in vivo studies on laboratory animals, which subsequently will allow proceeding to clinical tests. Polyphenolic compounds have a great potential as active ingredients to be used for the creation of new antiviral pharmaceutical substances.

Keywords: polyphenols; flavonoids; antioxidants; marine algae; anti-viral activity; mechanism of action

1. Introduction

The high virulence of new and recurring viruses and the lack of effective treatments for the diseases caused by them pose a serious challenge to public health systems. The development of highly effective broad-spectrum antiviral drugs with low toxicity and low cost has been one of the major issues in virology and pharmaceutics for many years. In the period of the ongoing COVID-19 pandemic, it has acquired particular relevance and importance and is aimed at creating agents that inhibit the entry and replication of the virus while modulating the body's defence systems.

The virus reproduction process includes three phases [1]. The first one is adsorption and entry of the virus into the cell, the release of its internal structural components, and modification into a state in which it can cause an infectious process. The attachment of the virus to macroorganism host cells is a specific interaction between the surface proteins of the virus and the receptors located on the surface of host cells. The second phase of reproduction is regulated by complex processes with the expression of the viral genome.

Finally, the third stage of reproduction is the release of viral offspring out of the host cell by budding or lysis.

Currently, medicine has a large range of antiviral agents that can have an effect on each of these stages [2]. At the same time, a rapid increase in their number is observed annually due to compounds isolated from terrestrial plants. The possibility of using synthetic and herbal preparations for the treatment of viral diseases is determined by a number of properties, such as a therapeutic effect, the absence or minimum of side reactions, and low toxicity.

Synthetic antiviral drugs act faster and provide, as a rule, the maximum therapeutic effect. However, their disadvantage is a large number of contraindications and side reactions, as well as addiction and the absence of the desired effect in the future. Herbal antiviral drugs have a wide spectrum of action (apart from the antiviral effect, they have anti-inflammatory, antioxidant and immunomodulatory effects), are less toxic or non-toxic in working doses, and have minimal side effects. It is possible that herbal medicine may have potential as a prophylactic agent and even a therapeutic agent for patients with viral infection.

Despite certain advances in chemotherapy of viral diseases, clinical practice faces serious problems such as the emergence of drug-resistant variants of viruses and side effects of antiviral medicines. This circumstance dictates the need to develop new antiviral drugs with different mechanisms of action [3,4].

Studies on compounds with antiviral properties derived from terrestrial and marine plants have shown that, due to their diverse mechanisms of action (antiviral, immunostimulatory, anti-inflammatory and antioxidant), viruses, as a rule, do not acquire resistance to these compounds. Therefore, aquatic organisms producing substances that are sometimes not found in terrestrial plants and have extremely high polyvalent biological activity have attracted the special attention of researchers [5].

The world's experience in using marine-derived pharmaceuticals shows the enormous potential of marine organisms as raw materials for the creation of original pharmaceutical substances and medicines [6]. Algae, sponges, bacteria, fungi, invertebrates, soft corals, fish, etc. can be sources of new antiviral pharmacological compounds of marine origin [7–9]. A number of compounds from these organisms are commercially available on the pharmaceutical market worldwide as an alternative to antiviral drugs [10].

The purpose of this review is to summarise the literature data on the antiviral potential of polyphenolic compounds of seaweed, to highlight the mechanisms of their action and to characterise the other biological properties of these compounds that affect the course and outcome of viral infections. The authors draw the attention of researchers to the fact that algae are an extremely promising source of antiviral compounds, and research in this direction should be continued.

2. General Characteristics of the Polyphenolic Compounds of Seaweed

Marine macroalgae are a unique raw material for obtaining a wide range of natural compounds with interesting and useful biological properties. Their composition is characterised by a rich content of mineral and organic substances. For thousands of years, these hydrobionts have been actively used by humans and animals for food and have served as a valuable source of proteins, fats, carbohydrates, dietary fibre, minerals, etc.

Regular consumption of seaweed can reduce the risk of various pathologies, including cancer, metabolic and degenerative disorders, infectious diseases and cardiovascular diseases. The highest antiviral activity, as shown by numerous experimental studies, is possessed by polyphenolic compounds and sulphated polysaccharides. The content of biologically active substances in seaweed varies depending on the season and region of collection and is largely determined by the type of algae. According to the presence of specific pigments, macroalgae are divided into three main groups: brown (Phaeophyceae), green (Chlorophyta) and red (Rhodophyta) seaweed.

Polyphenols (PPs)—highly hydrophilic secondary metabolites of seaweed—are one of the most numerous groups of substances in the plant kingdom. Macro- and microalgae, as well as cyanobacteria accumulate PPs, in particular, phloroglucinol and its polymers, i.e., phlorotannins [11]. Bromophenols, phenolic acids and flavonoids account for the largest proportion of phenolic compounds found in red and green seaweed [12]. Phlorotannins (PTs) are a heterogeneous group of unique polyphenolic compounds differing in structure and degree of polymerisation and are found only in brown seaweed (up to 25% of dry weight) [13,14]. The largest amount of PTs accumulates in fucus brown seaweed [15–18]. PTs consist of monomeric units of phloroglucinol (1,3,5-hydroxybenzene), from which more than 700 natural variations of these compounds have been obtained and used in various fields [19] (Figure 1).

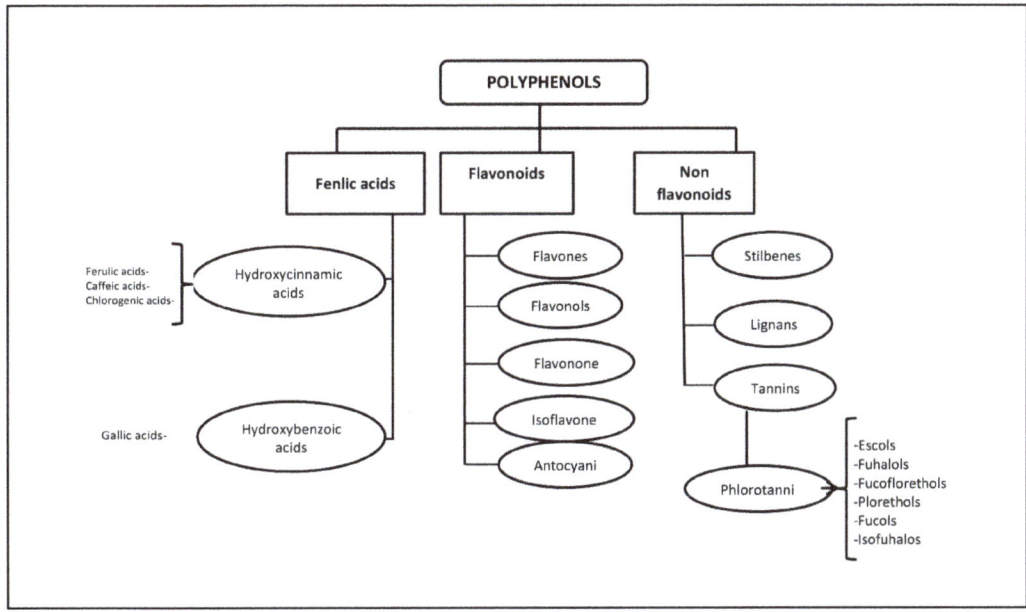

Figure 1. Classification of polyphenols and six main subclasses of seaweed phlorotannins.

Unlike the tannins of terrestrial plants, PTs have a wider range of molecular weights, from 126 Da to 650 kDa (more often from 10 to 100 kDa). The characterisation of PPs is difficult due to heterogeneity both in molecular weight and in the level of isomerisation [20,21]. There is still little information about endogenous digestion and microbial catabolism of these compounds [22]. It is known that about 90–95% of dietary PPs reach the intestine unchanged [23], where, as a result of metabolism and biotransformation, low molecular weight compounds with less chemical heterogeneity are formed than in the original [24].

Some PTs in seaweed can be sulphated or halogenated [25]. The biosynthesis of PTs is carried out through the acetate-malonate pathway in the Golgi apparatus in the perinuclear region of the cell. They are usually not secreted, and cell destruction is necessary to obtain them. In terms of structure and polymeric properties, PTs represent an extensive group of molecules that differ in the nature of the bonds between phloroglucinol and hydroxyl groups (Figure 1). Depending on the type of bond between the monomers, phlorotannins are divided into four subclasses: phlorethols and fuhalols, fucols, fucophlorethols, and eckols and carmalol [26,27]. These compounds exist mainly in a soluble form or in a bound state with components of the cell wall, which ensure its integrity as well as protection from herbivores and oxidative stress.

Terrestrial plants produce tannins that are composed of only three or four phenolic rings, while seaweed PTs are composed of eight phenolic rings. PTs have very strong antioxidant properties as phenolic rings act as electron traps for free radicals [12]. A positive correlation has been noted between the antioxidant activity of PTs and the number of hydroxyl groups present in the structure of the compound [28]. PTs inhibit α-glucosidase, which is responsible for the stepwise removal of terminal glucose residues from the N-glycan chains associated with glycoprotein maturation. Most glycoproteins of the viral environment contain N-linked glycans, and α-glucosidase inhibitors have been proposed as useful broad-spectrum antiviral agents based on their activity against enveloped viruses [29]. The anti-inflammatory [30], antiallergic [31], antiviral [32] and antitumor [33] properties, as well as antidiabetic and radioprotective effects [34] of these biologically active compounds have been demonstrated.

Methods for obtaining PTs, their identification and establishment of the structure are described in sufficient detail in numerous works [13,14,35]. The main difficulty in the extraction of PPs arises from their presence in the form of complex polymer mixtures, for example, with polysaccharides, which, along with proteins, are the main covalently bound component of the algal cell wall [36].

3. Interaction of Seaweed Polyphenols with Enveloped and Nonenveloped Viruses

Resistance of viruses to adverse environmental factors is determined by their structure. There are viruses with simple and complex structure. Simple, or nonenveloped, viruses are composed of a nucleic acid and protein envelope (capsid). Complex, or enveloped, viruses are surrounded by a lipoprotein envelope (supercapsid) over the capsid, which makes them more vulnerable to adverse environmental factors [5,6,23].

Enveloped and nonenveloped viruses also differ in resistance to chemicals, including disinfectants. Thus, the lipoprotein-enveloped influenza, parainfluenza viruses and coronaviruses are low-resistant pathogens; adenoviruses are more resistant; and the nonenveloped rhinovirus is one of the very resistant pathogens such as poliovirus and hepatitis A virus [37].

A. Interaction of Polyphenols of Seaweed with Enveloped Viruses

In recent years, intensive studies of the antiviral activity of polyphenolic compounds from terrestrial plants, as well as from various marine aquatic organisms, including macroalgae, have been carried out [38–41]. Mainly enveloped viruses are reported as sensitive to PPs. Figure 2 shows the targets of the enveloped virus that can be affected by plant polyphenols.

Tannins are known as powerful protein inactivators, including viral ones. M. Wink [38,39] showed that plant tannins form several hydrogen and ionic bonds when interacting with a virus protein, which act on the three-dimensional structure of the protein, suppressing its activity. As land plant tannins and algal tannins are similar in structure, the mechanisms of their interaction with enveloped viruses are probably similar. Polyphenols bind to viral envelope proteins, preventing the pathogen from interacting with the host cell.

Coronaviruses are enveloped viruses. To date, 39 known species of enveloped viruses are known, with each species comprising dozens and hundreds of strains. In addition to the nucleic acid and the associated structurally protective protein (in coronaviruses, it is the N protein), they also have a membrane envelope. The life cycle of coronaviruses provides many potential targets for antiviral intervention. Approaches to the development of anti-coronavirus drugs include exposure to the virus during the steps of penetration and entry of a viral particle into a cell, replication of viral nucleic acid, release of virion from a cell and effects on the cellular targets of the host.

One of the members of coronaviruses is the porcine epidemic diarrhoea virus (PEDL). First recorded in the United States in 2013, it has caused major economic damage in many countries due to the significant mortality of newborn piglets. The PEDL infects the cells lining the pig's small intestine, causing severe epidemic diarrhoea and dehydration [40,41].

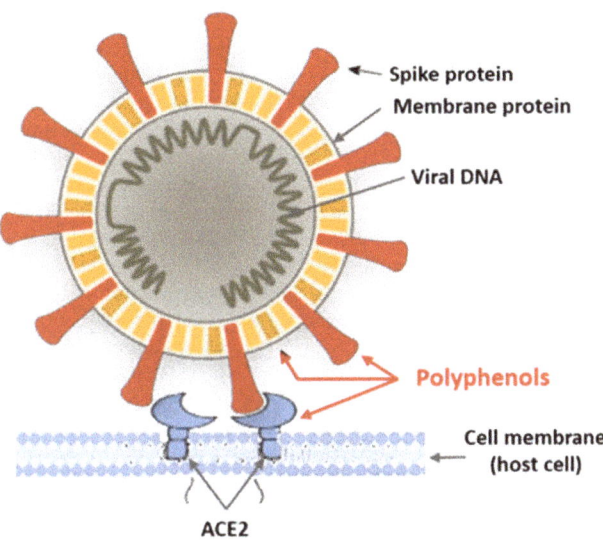

Figure 2. Targets of the enveloped virus for polyphenols of marine and terrestrial plants.

The causative agent was investigated using electron and immunoelectron microscopy. It was shown to differ from the coronaviruses known by that time: the porcine transmissible gastroenteritis (TGS) virus and porcine hemagglutinating encephalomyelitis. Kwon et al. [42] found an antiviral effect of ethanol extract and five phlorotannins obtained from the brown alga *Ecklonia cava* against the PEDL. The extracted compounds were identified as phloroglucinol (1), eckol (2), 7-phloreckol (3), phlorofucofuroeckol (4) and dieckol (5). Compounds (4) and (5) were present in the ethanol extract from seaweed in sufficiently large amounts [29].

To assess the antiviral activity of the compounds in vitro, two strategies were used: blocking the virus' binding to cells (obtaining the effect of treatment simultaneously with the infection) and inhibiting the virus' replication (obtaining the effect of treatment after the infection). The use of the former experimental scheme made it possible to establish that compounds (2–5) have an antiviral activity against the PEDL with the 50% inhibitory concentration (IC_{50}) in the range from 10.8 ± 1.4 to 22.5 ± 2.2 µM. Compounds (2–5) completely blocked the binding of virus protein to sialic acid at concentrations lower than 36.6 µM by inhibiting hemagglutination. The results of the use of the latter experimental design showed that these compounds also blocked the virus' replication with IC50 values of 12.2 ± 2.8 and 14.6 ± 1.3 µM, respectively, by inhibiting the synthesis of RNA and virus protein, but did not suppress the viral protease [28,30,31]. Regarding the cytotoxicity of the extract, the CC_{50} was 533.6 µg/mL and ranged from 374.4 to 579 µM for compounds (4) and (5). The experiments were carried out using the lowest toxic (>90% cell viability) concentrations of the extract [30,31].

The PT activity was distributed as follows: dieckol (16.6 ± 3.0 µM) > 7 phlorofucofuroeckol (18.6 ± 2.3 µM) > eckol (22.5 ± 2.3 µM). Phloroglucinol was inactive. PT activity was distributed as follows: dieckol (16.6 ± 3.0 µM) > 7 phlorofucofuroeckol (18.6 ± 2.3 µM) > eckol (22.5 ± 2.3 µM). Phloroglucinol was inactive. PT activity was influenced by the number of hydroxyl groups. Thus, oligomerisation and the existence of the cyclopentane ring may be important for the manifestation of antiviral activity. The authors recommend phlorofucofuroeckol and dieckol from the brown seaweed *E. cava* as potential agents that act on the most important targets of PEDV.

B. Interaction of PTs of Algae with Nonenveloped Viruses

However, enveloped viruses are not only sensitive to the action of plant phenolic compounds, in particular tannins. Ueda et al. [43] found, for example, that persimmon extracts containing about 22% tannin reduced the infectivity of nonenveloped viruses (poliovirus, Coxsackie virus, adenovirus, rotavirus, feline calcivirus and mouse norovirus) by more than 4 log. The authors believe that the main mechanism of the antiviral action of the extract is associated with the aggregation of viral proteins, as evidenced by the competitive suppression of the antiviral effect by BSA. Algal phlorotannins also have an inhibitory effect on nonenveloped viruses. Such results are noted for human papillomavirus (HPV). As an example, we consider HPV, a small, nonenveloped virus possessing a capsid with cubic symmetry and containing two proteins, L1 and L2. The former is the main capsid protein that makes up more than 80% of the capsid material, forming blocks (capsomeres) from which the capsid is built. Anti-L1 antibodies exhibit virus-neutralising activity. L2 is a minor protein involved in the capsid stabilisation and linking with the genome [44]. The genital infection caused by the human papillomavirus (HPV) is the most common sexually transmitted disease. Most cases of cervical cancer are associated with this infection. Therefore, there is considerable interest in new effective non-reactogenic drugs for the treatment and prevention of this disease.

Kim and Kwak [44] investigated the effect of PT from the brown alga *E. bicyclis* on HPV. It was found that the seaweed EtOH extract exhibited antiviral activity against HPV 16PVs and HPV 18PVs. Then, the extract was sequentially separated with CH_2Cl_2, EtOAc and n-BuOH. The most active EtOAc fraction was used for chromatographic separation and resulted in the isolation of eckol, 8,8′-bieckolm 6,6′-bieckol and phlorofucofuroeckol A-Antiviral activity was assessed in 293T cell culture using bioluminescence. All compounds showed a decrease in the viral load of both viruses at a concentration of 50 µg/mL.

Noroviruses, a nonenveloped type of enterovirus, are considered the leading cause of epidemics of diseases accompanied by vomiting, diarrhoea, mild fever, abdominal cramps and nausea [45,46]. Norovirus is characterised by a long isolation period, low infectious dose, high resistance, considerable diversity and frequent genome mutations. The virus is transmitted through contaminated water or food and is spread by the faecal–oral route following contact with infected materials. The virus has a single-stranded positive sense RNA genome [47]. In recent years, attempts have been made to find harmless means of therapy and prevention of infection among terrestrial and marine organisms and algae [48]. To this aim, Eom et al. [40] investigated the possibility of using *E. bicyclis* seaweed extract and its ingredients as an alternative agent against norovirus. The following fractions were obtained from the EtOAc-soluble extract of *E. bicyclis*: phlorofucofuroeckol A (PFE) and dieckol (DE).

The MeOH extract and its components did not show significant cytotoxicity. The CC_{50} was 322.48 to 2146.42 µg/mL. The EtOAc extract showed strong antiviral activity and low cytotoxicity. Earlier [40], the authors described the structure of the extract components DE and PFE and their pronounced antiviral properties. PFE inhibits norovirus infection more intensely than DE. The selective index (SI) values for DE and PFE were approximately 20- and 25-fold higher than that of green tea epigallocatechin gallate. The antiviral activity of DE at IC_{50} was 0.9 ± 0.06, SI—CC_{50} IC_{50}—550.6 ± 6.09; PFE, IC_{50}—0.9 ± 0.07, SI—668.87 ± 73.06 [49].

The results obtained by the authors indicate that the use of PTs from *E. bicyclis* seaweed against norovirus infection is promising. They suggested that PTs prevent viruses from attaching to host cells and proposed to conduct an in-depth study of the mechanisms of anti-rotavirus action of these compounds.

An extract and PTs (eckol and PFE) from the seaweed *E. cava* were used to enhance protection against the nonenveloped RNA haemorrhagic septicaemia virus (VHSV) causing a highly contagious disease of freshwater and marine fish at different ages [41]. Using cell culture from fathead minnow, it was found that the extract and PTs at low concentrations exhibited strong antiviral activity. When cells were treated with the extract and PT simultaneously with the infection, the values increased (46.4–96.4%) as compared with those in the variants of the experiment before (16.5–48.4%) and after the infection (39.5–56, five%). The IC$_{50}$ for the extract, eckol and PFE were 4.76 µM, 1.97 µM and 0.99 µM, respectively. The effect increased depending on the time of exposure. In in vivo experiments, a seaweed extract, administered orally at different doses to VHSV-infected flounder, increased the survival rate of fish (by 31.57% at a dose of 500 µg/g/day; by 12.5% at 50 µg/g/day) 12.5%) [40].

Thus, not only enveloped, but also nonenveloped viruses, are sensitive to seaweed PTs. The mechanism of action of these compounds towards the former is better known.

4. Seaweed Polyphenols and Their Inhibition of Vital Viral Proteins

An ideal antiviral agent should target the inhibition of key proteins involved in the pathogen's life cycle. Potential inhibitors of these structures of viruses are polyphenolic compounds of seaweed, and, in particular, PTs.

Currently, the spread of the SARS-CoV-2 coronavirus is a serious public health problem, the solution of which requires the development of effective and harmless drugs. Coronavirus proteins are translated by one long polyprotein, from which two proteases are released: Mpro (major protease) and PLpro (papain-like protease). The active site of SARS-CoV 3CLpro contains a catalytic dyad consisting of Cys145 and His41, where a cysteine residue (Cys145) acts as a nucleophile and a histidine residue (His41) acts as a common acid base in the proteolytic process.

The central role of this protein in SARS-CoV replication has made it a major potential target for the development of antiviral drugs. Inhibition of this enzyme blocks SARS-CoV replication and enhances the antiviral response [50–52]. PLpro plays a role in the maturation and release of new viral particles from the cell, as well as in inhibiting the production of type 1 interferon synthesised by cells for protection. Suppression of interferon synthesis occurs by the action of PLpro on the ISG-15 gene in cellular proteins [53].

As the SARS-CoV proteases (3-chymotrypsin-like protease 3CLpro and papain-like protease PLpro) are synthesised as large precursor proteins that are cleaved to form mature active proteins, and their structures are retained in all genera of coronaviruses, the substances targeted at these proteins may be an effective strategy for the treatment of coronavirus infection by suppressing the viral genome replication [53,54].

In recent years, a number of phenolic compounds have been isolated from terrestrial plants, with inhibitory activity against the PLpro of coronaviruses, with inhibitory activity against S, the protein responsible for the fusion of the virus and the host cell prior to its penetration, as well as with inhibitory activity against replication pathogen [55–57]. However, even studies of polyphenolic compounds of terrestrial plants as anti-coronavirus agents, despite very encouraging results, are still at the experimental stage [58]. At the same time, the results of these studies allow researchers to hope that seaweed PPs may be more effective antiviral agents than polyphenols of terrestrial plants.

Park et al. [57], for the first time, studied PTs from the seaweed *E. cava* as an inhibitor of PLpro of the SARS-CoV virus. The authors obtained nine PTs from the ethanol extract from the seaweed. In the experiments using cell-free analysis, it was found that eight PTs (triphlorethol A, eckol, dioxinodehydroeckol, 2-phloreckol, 7-phloreckol, fucodiphlorethol, dieckol and phlorofucofuroeckol A) were dose-dependent competitive inhibitors of SARS-CoV 3CLpro. The IC$_{50}$ values varied from 2.7 ± 0.6 (dieckol) to 164.7 ± 10.8 µM (triphlorethol A). The best inhibitory effect was exhibited by dieckol, which has two eckol groups linked via diphenyl ether [57].

The PTs of seaweed interact with vital proteins of other viruses, in particular with influenza virus neuraminidase (NA). Neuraminidase and hemagglutinin of the pathogen determine the antigenic properties of this pathogen. Hemagglutinin initiates infection by binding of the virus to α-2,6-sialic acid and/or α-2,3-linked sialic acid receptors on the host cell surface, followed by receptor-mediated endocytosis into the cell [59]. The sialic acid receptor on the surface of the host cell is a commonly recognised target for the development of broad-spectrum antiviral agents. Sialidase hydrolyses sialic acid on the cell surface and prevents the virus from attaching to cells. The NA protein serves as a sialidase and cleaves the bond between sialic acid and the HA protein to release virus particles. Neuraminidase thus plays a critical role in the life cycle of the influenza virus and also serves as an attractive target for the development of anti-influenza drugs [59]. PTs of seaweed can be used as candidates for the creation of such preparations.

Algae-derived PTs are considered candidates for such agents. In their work, Cho et al. [44] studied PTs from the seaweed *E. cava*, which is widely used as food in Asian countries, in particular Japan and Korea. Its main components are phlorotannins and fucoidan [60]. The authors investigated the antiviral activity against the influenza virus of 13 PTs obtained from 80% MeOH-extract of algae, which contained in their structures at least one fragment of 1,4-dibenzodioxin and were found mainly in Ecklonia and some other species seaweed [61,62]. Phlorofucofuroeckol A at IC_{50} = 13.48 ± 1.93 µM showed the highest antiviral activity against two strains of influenza A virus (H1N1 and H9N2). Six PTs showed a sufficiently high or moderate antiviral activity against both virus strains at a concentration of 20 µM. The compounds with high antiviral activity were tested for the synthesis of the viral protein of the H1N1A/PR/8/34 virus compared that of ribavirin as a positive control. Phlorofucofuroeckol A was tested on Madin–Darby canine kidney (MDCK) cells at concentrations of 5, 10, 20 and 40 µM. The compound more effectively inhibited viral protein expression in infected cells. In addition, this phlorotannin reduced the expression of NA and HA at a dose of 10 µM, and its strongest inhibitory activity was observed at a dose of 40 µM.

In the work of Ryu et al. [63], an ethanol extract from *E. cava* was fractionated, and five PTs were isolated. The extract showed a strong anti-neuraminidase activity (71.1% inhibition at a dose of 30 µg/mL). The inhibitory activity was studied on various strains of the influenza virus. Eckol showed a moderate IC_{50} value (89.5 µM) against the influenza A/Bervig-Mission/1/18 (H1N1) virus, but was inactive towards other viral strains (IC_{50} > 200 µM) compared to the other compounds tested (7-phloreckol, phlorofucofuroeckol, and dieckol). The IC_{50} value of the compounds increased with an increase in the number of hydroxyl groups (from eckol to dieckol), which indicates the significance of this trait in NA inhibition. All the studied PTs were selective NA inhibitors [63].

Thus, phlorofucofuroeckol A from brown seaweed *E. cava* plays a key role in the antiviral activity of these algae against influenza viruses H1N1 and H9N2 and may be the basis for the further development of anti-influenza drugs, dietary supplements for food and functional food products.

Acquired immunodeficiency syndrome (AIDS) caused by the human immunodeficiency virus (HIV) is a major public health problem worldwide, especially in developing countries [64]. The human immunodeficiency virus (HIV) belongs to the family Retroviridae and the genus *Lentivirus*. It is an RNA enveloped virus with an unusual method of replication of genetic material. *Lentiviruses* (in Latin, "lente" means "slowly") can cause diseases with a long incubation period and a slow, but steady progressive course. The cycle of their reproduction is characterised by a reverse flow of genetic information, i.e., DNA synthesis is carried out on a viral RNA matrix using an enzyme, reverse transcriptase (RT). RT, being vitally important for the virus, is a heterodimer (a protein of two polypeptide chains), consisting of two subunits (p66 and p51) [64].

Currently, the following antiviral drugs that act on various targets of the virus are available: nucleoside RT inhibitors, non-nucleoside RT inhibitors, protease inhibitors, integrase inhibitors, fusion inhibitors and antagonists of chemokine receptors (Table 1).

Unfortunately, HIV resistance to drugs is increasing daily; in addition, many of these agents have adverse side effects. For this reason, scientists' attention has been attracted by new-generation drugs, to which HIV would not form resistance. Noteworthy and promising results were obtained in a study of anti-HIV properties of algae-derived PTs.

Table 1. Antiretroviral drugs that act on various targets of the virus.

Antiviral Drug Class	Antiviral Mechanism of Action	Examples of Available Drugs
Nucleoside/nucleotide reverse transcriptase inhibitors (NRTIs)	Affect the ability of a virus to multiply or reproduce. NRTIs prevent the virus's reverse transcriptase from accurately copying its RNA into DNA.	Zidovudine (Retrovir), Lamivudine (Epivir), Abacavir sulfate (Ziagen), Didanosine (Videx), Stavudine (Zerit), Emtricitabine (Emtriva)
Non-nucleoside reverse transcriptase inhibitors (NNRTIs)	NNRTIs block DNA elongation by directly binding to the reverse transcriptase enzyme	Delavirdine, Efavirenz, Etravirine, Nevirapine, Rilpivirine
Protease inhibitors	Protease inhibitor drugs block the action of protease enzymes. This can stop the virus from multiplying.	Atazanavir (Reyataz), Darunavir (Prezista), Fosamprenavir (Lexiva), Indinavir (Crixivan), Nelfinavir (Viracept), Ritonavir (Norvir), Saquinavir (Invirase)
Integrase inhibitors	These drugs stop HIV from being able to make integrase, which is necessary for its replication.	Raltegravir (Isentress), Dolutegravir (Tivicay), Elvitegravir, Bictegravir
Inhibitors of fusion	Inhibitors of the fusion of HIV to host cells, preventing viral entry.	Enfuvirtide, Maraviroc, Leronlimab, Aplaviroc, Ibalizumab, Temsavir
Inhibitors of chemokine receptors	These drugs inhibit chemokine receptors (CXCR4 and CCR5) and block the entry virus into the host cell.	Selzentry (Pro) Maraviroc, Bicyclam derivatives, AMD070

Ahn et al. [65] showed that 8,8-bieckol and 8,4 dieckol from the brown alga *E. cava* inhibit reverse transcriptase and HIV-1 protease, while eckol and phlorofucofuroeckol A from this alga did not exhibit such activity. 8,8-Bieckol and 8,4 dieckol more efficiently inhibited RT than protease. The IC_{50} of dieckol towards RT was 0.51 µM and was comparable to that of a reference drug, nevirapine (IC_{50} = 0.28 µM) [65]. 8,8-Bieckol and 8,4 dieckol more efficiently inhibited RT than protease. The IC_{50} of dieckol towards RT was 0.51 µM and was comparable to that of a reference drug, nevirapine (IC_{50} = 0.28 µM) [65]. Furthermore, the authors obtained diphlorethohydroxycarmalol, a carmalol derivative, from the marine brown alga *Ishige okamurae*. This compound had an inhibitory effect on RT and HIV-1 integrase with IC_{50} values of 9.1 µm and 25.2 µm, respectively. However, this compound did not have the same effect on HIV-1 protease. Acetylation neutralised this effect. 6,6′-Bieckol from *E. cava* reduced the cytopathic effects of HIV-1, including HIV-1-induced syncytium formation and p24 antigen levels.

Artan et al. [66] isolated 6,6′-bieckol, a phloroglucinol derivative, from the alga *E. cava* and characterised the compound by NMR. This phlorotannin showed a strong inhibition of HIV-1-induced syncytium formation (IC_{50} = 1.72 µM), viral p24 antigen production (IC_{50} = 1.26 µM) and lytic effects (IC_{50} = 1.23 µM). The compound selectively inhibited the activity of HIV-1 reverse transcriptase at IC_{50} = 1.07 µM, as well as the entry of HIV into cells. The authors proposed 6,6′-dieckol as a candidate for a new-generation drug against HIV infection [66].

Additionally, Karadeniz et al. [67] reported the anti-HIV activity of 8,4′-dieckol, a phloroglucinol derivative of *E. cava*. The compound dose-dependently inhibited the cytopathogenic effects of HIV-1, including HIV-1-induced syncytium formation in C8166 cells; suppressed lytic effects; and reduced the production of the viral p24 protein by H9 cells. Like the above-described agents, 8,4′-dieckol inhibited reverse transcriptase and viral penetration. However, it was found that, over time, the amount of syncytium in infected C8166 cells increased, the inhibitory activity was lost and phlorotannin had to be reintroduced into the cell culture [67].

It is important to emphasise that this compound suppressed replication of a virus with resistance to three drugs when cells were treated within 6 h post-infection. Similar results were obtained for nevirapine, the reverse transcriptase inhibitor. The authors suggest that the studied phlorotannin exhibits the effect of HIV-1 reverse transcriptase inhibition, possibly due to the binding of RT to sites or conformations other than those of virapine. This phlorotannin is a promising drug for the further development of new agents against HIV-1 with a pronounced efficacy compared to drugs available on the market [68]. Thus, using the example of three pathogens of most widespread viral infections, we have shown algal PTs to be promising for the creation of anti-HIV drugs whose targets are enzymes vital for viruses. In addition, these compounds also inhibit such viral functions as replication, entry in cell, syncytium formation, etc.

Note, however, that the degree of bioavailability of PT and individual differences in metabolism are significant limitations of their use. In addition, there are currently no analytical standards for the study of PT, and the exact relationship between the structure of compounds and their bioactivity is also unclear [67,68]. The authors suggest that the efficacy of medicinal plants against COVID-19 is not yet sufficiently demonstrated by studies, although some of them exhibiting IC_{50} below 10 µM can be considered promising, as they are capable of blocking viral proteins associated with its life cycle. After obtaining clinical evidence of the useful properties of algal PTs, these compounds in the form of natural products or biologically active substances can be combined with approved drugs against pathogenic viruses, which may be a promising alternative for the prevention and treatment of infections caused by them [68].

5. Synergism of Algae-Derived Phlorotannins and Antiviral Drugs

In viral infections, the simultaneous effect of drugs on several targets of the causative agent is of great importance, and therefore combined therapy has a number of advantages that allow:

- reduction in individual doses of drugs;
- reduction in the number and severity of side effects of antiviral drugs; and
- prevention, in some cases, of the emergence of drug-resistant virus variants [69].

The combination of targeted technologies with the inclusion of natural biologically active substances in the treatment regimen has shown numerous advantages of this therapeutic approach.

Although measles is a controllable infection, it takes thousands of children's lives each year even in developed countries, and therefore the search for new natural compounds for the prevention and treatment of this infection continues. Moran-Santibanez et al. [70] investigated the effectiveness of the combined use of seaweed extracts rich in PPs and sulphated polysaccharides derived from the same seaweed and ribavirin against the measles virus. The authors used extracts from two seaweeds, *Ecklonia arborea* (class Phaeophyceae) and *Solieria filiformis* (phylum Rhodophyta), in experiments on a line of African green monkey kidney cells (Vero). Both extracts were characterised by low toxicity, high (compared with ribavirin) antiviral activity and high selectivity index (>3750 and >576.9, respectively). The selectivity index is the ratio of the 50% toxic concentration of a drug to its 50% virus-inhibiting concentration [70].

The extraction was carried out in accordance with the method described by Xi et al. [71] with six (*Ecklonia*) and five (*Solieria*) fractions obtained from the extracts. Phlorofucofuroeckol A was obtained from *E. arborea*. All samples used in the experiments were non-toxic to cells at the concentrations tested (from 0.1 to 1500 µg/mL). Ribavirin exhibited cytotoxicity starting with the 50% cytotoxic concentration (CC_{50}) = 405 µg/mL.

All the tested components exhibited antiviral activity, which was assessed by determining the decrease in syncytium formation at various concentrations of the compounds (0.01, 0.1, 1 and 5 µg/mL of each extract and 10, 20, 30, 40 and 5 µg/mL ribavirin).

The combined effect was also assessed by determining the reduction in the syncytium formation. A combination of PT from *Ecklonia* and *S. filiformis* with sulphated polysaccharides (SPS) from *Solieria* showed the best synergistic effects, which was confirmed by PCR analysis. The best result was obtained by using PP from *Ecklonia* at IC_{50} and *Solieria* at IC_{25} + SPS from *Solieria*. All combinations with ribavirin were antagonistic. The authors noted that phlorotannins were most effective within the first 15 min post-infection, which suggests that this effect is due to direct inactivation of viral particles through preventing their adsorption and entry into cell.

The probability of viral entry into cells in the present of extracts was also determined. The best inhibitory effect was observed in the case of the *S. filiformis* extract compared to the control samples.

The virucidal activity of seaweed extracts is not only a preventive strategy to be implemented before a viral infection, but can also be an effective treatment after infection to prevent the virus from spreading over the body. Synergistic effect of ribavirin with PT with sulphated polysaccharides from the same seaweed can allow for a reduction in the concentration of drugs and thereby their cytotoxicity, as well as prevent the formation of resistance to therapeutic agents.

6. The Effect of PT on Pathogenetic Targets of Viral Infections in a Macroorganism

The role of the antioxidant properties of PT in the organism's defence against viruses: Oxidative stress induced by a viral infection plays a significant role in the pathogenesis of infectious diseases [72]. Oxidative stress disrupts the balance between the production of free radicals, including reactive oxygen species (ROS), and the signalling pathways of antioxidant cells. It is a key factor in the pathogenesis of many acute and chronic viral diseases [73,74].

Reactive oxygen species (ROS) (such as superoxide radical anion (O-), hydroxyl radical (HO-) and nitric oxide (NO) and potential endogenous prooxidants, such as hydrogen peroxide (H_2O_2), hydrochloric acid (HC10), peroxynitrite (NO_3^-) and lipo-hydroperoxide (MOOH), have high reactivity, which damages the proteins, nucleic acids and lipids of the biological membranes of cells. Oxidative stress is a key factor in signal transmission by inflammatory cells for the regulation of cytokines and growth factors, as well as for immunomodulation and apoptosis [75]. It is known that oxidative processes contribute to viral replication in infected cells [76] and have an effect on the inhibition of cell proliferation and induction of apoptosis [77]. Thus, in patients infected with herpes simplex virus [78], the increased peroxidation of membrane phospholipids, induced by ROS, causes dysfunction of vital cell processes such as membrane transport and mitochondrial respiration [79]. The green tea component epigallocatechin has been shown to block the entry of HIV [80] due to its antioxidant properties.

Chen et al. [80] reported that infections caused by the Epstein–Barr virus (EBV) cause an increase in DNA damage and a significant accumulation of ROS; however, the use of free radical scavengers reduced the intensity of damage both in cells stimulated by the mitogen and in cells infected by this virus. A suggestion has been made that antioxidants counteract the damaging effects of reactive oxygen and nitrogen species, including free radicals, and therefore prevent or have a therapeutic effect on diseases associated with oxidative stress [81].

Modern medicine seeks to use various antioxidants to combat oxidative stress in viral infections. There is much evidence for the ability of natural antioxidants to trap ROS in infected cells, inhibit proapoptotic factors and thus restore intracellular balance between stress-related proteins (N-terminal kinases with Jun-JNK0 and promitotic (MAPK) and transcription factors NF-kB) [82–84]. Seaweeds are a rich source of antioxidants including PTs [76].

Viruses can be the causative agents of neuroinfections, directly mediating oxidative stress, the central link of which is the peroxidation of lipids, which play a key role in the nervous system [72]. Thus, the beneficial properties of phlorotanins are associated with their properties as a powerful antioxidant, anti-inflammatory and immunoregulatory molecule, as well as with their neuroprotective effect.

In neurotropic flavivirus infections (such as JEV, WNV and TBEV infections), oxidative stress is an important component of neuroinflammation [85,86]. When various neuronal cell lines were infected with flaviviruses, the increase in ROS production induced uncontrolled activation of microglia and neuronal death [87]. Being ROS scavengers, polyphenolic compounds from seaweeds are considered as potent antioxidants. In this regard, the polyphenolic complex luromarin derived from the seagrass *Zostera marina*, containing phenolpropanoid and flavone, is of great interest. Note that phenolpropanoid, in terms of antioxidant activity, is noticeably superior to all known antioxidants [85–87].

Studies [88] have provided data on in vitro and in vivo studies of the antiviral efficacy of a PP complex isolated from seagrasses of the family Zosteraceae, which are flowering plants adapted to living in saline water of seas and oceans.

The antiviral activity of luromarin and its components against a highly virulent strain of tick-borne encephalitis (TBE) virus was studied in vitro. It was found that the exposure to these compounds at 1 h before the infection of the cells had no effect on the reproduction of the virus. A different result was obtained by the authors in the study of direct virucidal action (preliminary incubation of the compounds under study with the virus for 1 h before cell infection) [89–91]. Thus, the main mechanism of action of the natural antioxidants (that make up luromarin) and the entire complex against the TBE virus is the direct inactivation of viral particles and inhibition of the TBE virus at an early stage of replication.

In a model of acute TBE infection in mice, oral administration of luromarin and its components at 1 h after subcutaneous infection of animals provided 30–35% protection by increasing their lifespan by 2–3 days compared to the control. The authors explain this by the complex protective effect of luromarin and its components, which have not only a selective effect on various phases of viral infection, but also a systemic effect on the body due to their high antioxidant, anti-inflammatory and neuroprotective potential.

The Role of Anti-Inflammatory Action of Polyphenols in Protection against Viral Infections

Inflammation is a complex process regulated by a cascade of various proinflammatory cytokines, growth factors, nitric oxide and prostaglandins produced by activated macrophages [92]. With inflammation, the affected tissues become infiltrated by macrophages, and the disposal of decay products, repair and regeneration occur. The anti-inflammatory effect of phenolic compounds is directly related to their antioxidant activity against ROS [93].

The cytokine production and secretion are among the earliest events accompanying the interaction of microorganisms with macrophages. This early non-specific response to infection is important for the organism. It develops very quickly, as it does need a clone of cells that respond to a specific antigen. The early cytokine response influences the subsequent specific immune response.

The contact of a virus with an organism is accompanied by the production of interferon, a soluble factor produced by virus-infected cells. Interferon is capable of inducing antiviral status in uninfected cells and makes them unsuitable for viral reproduction. Interferon activates macrophages which begin to synthesise IFN-γ, IL-1, IL-2, IL-4, IL-6 and TNF-α; as a result, macrophages acquire the ability to lyse cells infected by the virus. At the same time, interferon is able to induce expression of more than 100 different genes in the macrophage genome [94].

In some cases, e.g., in severe cases of coronavirus infection (COVID-19), a "cytokine storm" develops. It is an inflammatory response of organism, with the level of cytokines in blood increasing sharply, which causes the immunity to attack cells and tissues of own organism. A consequence of this response can be the destruction of tissues and organs and, as a result, the death of the organism.

Seaweed PPs are not only antiviral, but also potent anti-inflammatory compounds. For example, 8,8′-dieckol from the seaweed *E. cava* inhibited the production of nitric oxide, a key mediator of inflammation, and prostaglandin E2 (PGE2) by macrophages stimulated by lipopolysaccharide. This compound inhibited the production of nitric oxide by suppressing the expression of inducible nitric oxide synthesis (iNOS). Phlorotannin reduced the production and expression of IL-6 mRNA, but did not inhibit TNFα. The exposure of macrophages to this PT decreased the NF-κB transactivation and the nuclear translocation of the p65 NF-κB subunit and suppressed the lipopolysaccharides (LPS)-induced production of intracellular ROS in macrophages. Thus, the anti-inflammatory properties of PT are associated with the suppression of NO, PGE2 and IL-6 through the negative regulation of the NF-κB pathway and ROS production in RAW264 macrophages [95].

The range of anti-inflammatory effects may vary between different PTs. Thus, phlorofucofuroeckol A from the alga *Eisenia bicyclis* also exhibited an anti-inflammatory effect in the same model. In addition to reducing NO and PGE2, phlorotannin dose-dependently inhibited the production of COX-2 cyclooxygenase by macrophages, and also reduced the production of the proinflammatory chemokine MCP-1 [84]. These authors, as well as previous ones who worked with other PTs, showed that phlorofucofuroeckol A exerts an anti-inflammatory effect by blocking the NF-κB and MAPK signalling pathways in RAW264.7 macrophages stimulated by LPS. Eckol, a compound widely distributed in the brown seaweed *Ecklonia*, has attracted scientists' interest as an anti-inflammatory agent [96–98].

The inflammatory process is an inevitable consequence of viral infections. In this regard, algal PPs, which have both antiviral and anti-inflammatory effects, are promising objects for the development of drugs, biologically active food additives and functional food products on their basis.

7. In Vivo Efficacy of Polyphenolic Compounds

The results obtained under in vitro conditions are not always adequate to those obtained under the conditions of a macroorganism. For polyphenols, in many cases there is no direct correlation between the results of in vitro experiments and clinical trials, and the interpretation of experimental data should be treated with great caution.

Almost all in vitro experiments use flavonoid aglycones or polyphenol-rich extracts. In this regard, it can be assumed that under the conditions of a macroorganism, target organs almost never come into direct contact with aglycones of flavonoids, but only with their metabolites or conjugated forms [99,100]. In addition, the concentrations of aglycones that are commonly used in vitro experiments are almost never achieved in vivo. Therefore, after consumption of a single polyphenolic compound in doses of 10–100 mg, its maximum concentration in blood serum, as a rule, does not exceed 1 mM. Moreover, with rare exceptions, native flavonoids (aglycones) in the blood usually cannot be determined [99–102].

This section presents the results of an in vivo study of the antiviral activity of several polyphenolic compounds, which, according to other indications, are already used in medicine with positive effects in the form of medicines or biologically active food additives. They are presented by us as proof of the prospects of this group of biologically active substances for use as antiviral agents of a new generation with different mechanisms of action than synthetic drugs.

Quercetin and its derivatives: Quercetin, like other flavonoids, is a polyphenolic compound, the main structural element of which is composed of two aromatic rings, A and B, connected by a three-carbon bridge, forming a pyran or pyrone (in the presence of double bonds) ring [103]. This group of compounds has long attracted attention as potential therapeutic agents for the fight against respiratory tract infections [104].

Thus, Choi et al. [105] investigated the activity of quercetin-3 rhamnoside (Q3R) against the influenza A/WS/33 virus in mice. The animals received the drug orally (6.25 mg/kg per dose) two hours before infection and once a day for 6 days after infection with the influenza virus. In animals treated with Q3R, there was a significant reduction in weight loss and mortality. The titres of the virus in the lungs of mice in this group on day 6 after infection were about 2000 times lower than in animals treated with the control drug: oseltamivir. The use of the test drug delayed the development and progression of lung lesions. The authors believe that this compound may be a promising candidate for the development of anti-influenza drugs. As for the bioavailability of the compound, it is known that such derivatives are absorbed more efficiently than aglycone. A characteristic feature of the bioavailability of flavonols is their very slow elimination from the body (the half-life is from 11 to 28 h), which can contribute to the accumulation of metabolites in the blood plasma during repeated administration [106].

It was found that quercetin inhibits oxidative stress induced by the influenza virus [107]. The administration of quercetin to mice infected with the influenza A/Hong Kong/8/68 virus significantly reduced the level of lipid peroxidation in the animal body. In the lungs of such mice, the level of antioxidant enzymes—superoxide dismutase, catalase and reduced glutathione—increased [108]. Quercetin and rutin are recommended for inclusion in post-infection treatment [107,108].

To reduce the body's susceptibility to upper respiratory tract infections after stressful physical exertion, a short-term inclusion of quercetin in the diet is recommended, which has been proven by convincing results from in vivo studies [109].

The efficacy of quercetin has also been demonstrated in vivo experiments for respiratory tract infections caused by rhinovirus, which causes most colds and is a common cause of exacerbations in patients with asthma and chronic obstructive pulmonary disease [110,111]. The authors injected mice intranasally with the rhinovirus RV1B, which causes inflammation and interferon (IFN) production [112]. After 2 h, the animals were injected with quercetin or propylene glycol (vehicle). After a day and 4 days, the mice were sacrificed and the viral load in the lungs was determined, respectively. The viral load in animals infected with rhinovirus was 9×10^4 CC ID_{50}/mL of virus. No virus was detected after 4 days [112]. The mice treated with quercetin had a viral load that was 4 log less in the RNA of the virus compared to animals that received only the virus. In this case, the replication of the pathogen occurs only on the first day after infection and quercetin effectively inhibits this process. In addition, it helps to reduce the inflammatory process—it lowers the levels of CXCL-1 (KC), CXCL-2 (MIP-2), as well as TNFα and CCL2 (MCP-1). In mice not treated with quercetin, elevated levels of all four cytokines/chemokines were observed. The therapeutic effect was more pronounced when quercetin was used simultaneously or after infection.

Thus, quercetin suppresses rhinovirus-mediated viral infection at several stages of the viral life cycle, including endocytosis, viral genome transcription and viral protein synthesis; thus, it may be useful in limiting pathogen replication and reducing disease symptoms. Moreover, it is a powerful antioxidant and has powerful anti-inflammatory properties.

Enteroviruses pose a serious threat to human health. They cause a variety of pathological processes from mild disorders to death. The number of safe and effective drugs against enteroviruses is small, and therefore there is a need to develop new anti-enterovirus drugs. Galochkina et al. [113] investigated the effect of dihydroquercetin (DHQ) on the course of pancreatitis in white mice caused by Coxsackie B4 virus (CVB4). DHQ is a natural biologically active substance obtained from the bark of Siberian larch. It is a bioflavonoid with powerful antioxidant and anti-inflammatory properties. DHQ is on the drug registry and is non-toxic even at very high doses. The drug was administered to mice intraperitoneally at doses of 75 or 150 mg/kg/day once a day for 5 days after intraperitoneal infection. Ribavirin was used for comparison. The use of DHQ led to a dose-dependent decrease in the titre of the virus in the tissue of the pancreas. The morphology of the gland tissue of the animals receiving DHQ was less pronounced than in the control animals, displaying infiltration with inflammatory cells and no signs of destruction. The glandular tissue of mice treated with both DHQ and ribavirin had fewer inflammatory foci, and the latter, in turn, contained fewer infiltrating cells than animals treated with placebo. The effect was comparable to or superior to that of ribavirin. The authors concluded that DHQ is promising for use in the complex treatment of viral pancreatitis [113].

Another quercetin derivative, quercetin 3-β-O-D-glucoside, has been shown to be effective against the Ebola virus. This compound protected ABD2F1/Jena mice from intraperitoneal infection with Col.Sk, MM, MengoM, L viruses, but did not protect against intracerebral infection. The drug protected mice from Ebola even when administered just 30 min before infection, which allowed the authors to position the compound as having potential as a prophylactic agent against Ebola virus infection [114]. However, more serious research is required to finally determine the effectiveness of the compound for different modes of administration, different doses, etc.

Thus, a significant number of studies in vivo carried out both in animals and with the participation of patients show that quercetin is a promising candidate for combination therapy for various viral infections [115]. The above materials make it possible to consider the use of quercetin and its derivatives as promising for viral infections of various aetiologies. However, caution should be noted in extrapolating data from animals to humans [106].

Baikalin. The flavonoid baikalin is obtained from the roots of the *Scutellaria baicalensis*. In alternative medicine, it is used as a biologically active food supplement and in Asian countries as a drug. Currently, there is an extensive list of agents approved for use on the basis of or in combination with baikalin, the effectiveness of which has been proven for various indications in vivo. Many works carried out in vivo are devoted to the study of the effectiveness of baikalin in infections caused by different strains of the influenza virus [116–118].

Chu et al. [118] investigated in an experiment on mice the effect of baikalin on the human influenza A/PR/8/34 strain adapted to these animals. C57Bl/6 mice were inoculated with 0.1 LD_{50} (5×10^3 PFU/mL) of influenza virus. All infected mice died by day 8. Mice that received different doses of baikalin (1.0 g/kg, 1.5 g/kg and 2.0 g/kg) survived by day 8 (70%, 80% and 80%, respectively), and 60%, 70% and 80% survived until day 14, respectively. They did not lose weight. Virus titres in mice untreated with baikalin on day 7 increased to 106.3 pfu/mL. The titres of the virus in those who received the test preparation were, respectively, 102.7, 102.3 and 102.2 pfu/mL. Hemagglutination titres in untreated mice were 1:640, and in groups receiving the compound were 1:80, which indicates the inhibitory activity of baikalin on viral replication. Baikalin also inhibited the development of the inflammatory process in the lungs. In the same experiments, it was found that baikalin induces the secretion of IFNγ, which determines the antiviral activity of this compound. The last statement is proved by the fact that this compound did not have an antiviral effect in animals with IFNγ gene knockout [118].

In another study [119], it was found that oral administration of baikalin to mice infected with the Sendai virus leads to a significant reduction in virus titres in the lungs of animals and protection from death.

Resveratrol. Resveratrol is a highly active polyphenolic compound that is currently being actively studied both in vitro and in vivo as an antiviral agent [120,121]. The antiviral effects of this compound are associated with inhibition of viral replication, protein synthesis, gene expression and nucleic acid synthesis. The antioxidant effect of resveratrol is manifested by inhibiting important gene pathways such as NF-kB.

Resveratrol is poorly soluble in water and has a low oral bioavailability, and therefore research is currently focused on the development of structured nanoparticles that can improve the bioavailability of this biologically active substance and prolong its in vivo release.

Resveratrol has been used to prevent airway inflammation and reduce airway hypersensitivity caused by respiratory syncytial virus (RSV) infection. Healthy mice are immune to this pathogen. However, immunocompromised animals (treatment with cyclophosphamide) become susceptible to the virus [120]. It was found that resveratrol suppresses viral replication in the lungs of these mice and the number of infiltrating lymphocytes present in the lavage bronchoalveolar fluid reduces inflammation. In addition, resveratrol significantly reduced lavage fluid IFNγ levels associated with RSV-mediated airway inflammation [120].

In addition, resveratrol was highly active against rotavirus, which is the main causative agent of viral gastroenteritis in infants and young children [121]. Using a model of suckling mice infected with rotavirus, the authors found that resveratrol supplementation significantly reduced the severity of diarrhea, reduced viral titres and improved clinical symptoms. In the tissues of mice treated with resveratrol, the levels of expression of mRNA, IL-2, IL-10, TNFα, IFNγ, MIP-1 and MCP-1 were significantly reduced. Experiments have shown the promise of resveratrol as a potential treatment for rotavirus infection [121].

We have shown only some of the results of an in vivo study of the effectiveness of certain plant polyphenols known to all, on the basis of which approved drugs and biologically active food additives were obtained. Analysis of modern literature shows that these compounds are being actively studied now in vitro, ex vivo and in animal experiments. There are still very few clinical evidence-based studies on the effectiveness of this group of herbal biologically active substances. In this regard, the results obtained by Matsumoto et al. [122]. The authors conducted a double-blind, placebo-controlled study with 200 health workers conducted over 5 months at three health facilities for the elderly in Higashimuraami (Japan). One group of patients (98 people) received green tea catechins (378 mg/day) and theanine (210 mg/day). The control group (99 people) received a placebo. Four participants in the catechins/theanine group and 13 in the control group contracted the flu. Thus, the consumption of green tea catechins and theanine had a distinct preventive effect on the incidence of influenza.

Currently, polyphenolic compounds from land and sea plants are being actively studied due to their high biological activity. However, scientists must look for ways to increase the bioavailability of these compounds. For this purpose, many studies have proposed structural derivatives of the starting compounds. Some studies suggest using nanoparticles to encapsulate polyphenolic compounds for greater efficacy. In addition, the administration of polyphenolic compounds with other antiviral drugs can improve their bioavailability. An example is the studies of O'Shea et al. [123]. The authors examined the efficacy of monoclonal antibodies (mAb; AR4A) and epigallocatechin gallate (EGCG) in vitro and in vivo. The combination therapy completely protected animals from HCV 1a genotype infection.

Regarding new polyphenolic compounds, which are currently being studied in large numbers all over the world, serious studies of their specificity, activity, bioavailability and safety are required before they are proposed as drugs. After careful testing and approval for use in humans, it can be recommended to use such compounds in the form of dietary supplements and nutritional supplements.

It is necessary to develop strategies for increasing the bioavailability of polyphenols, to determine whether these methods lead to an increase in biological activity in the body. The benefits and efficacy of polyphenols in viral infections should be demonstrated in appropriate animal and human disease models.

8. Conclusions

PPs are unique compounds found in seaweed at high concentrations. For example, *Ascophyllum nodosum* contains 14% PPs, compared to 2–3% in terrestrial plants. The high concentration of PPs in seaweed, combined with the simplicity of their cultivation, harvesting and processing, makes them attractive as a cheap source of pharmaceutical substances and a basis for creating dietary supplements for food and functional foods.

Algae-derived PPs (phlorotannins) combine several types of activities, each of which contributes to decrease in viral load, decrease in the intensity of the inflammatory process, increase in the antioxidant properties of blood and correction of immune disorders. It has been shown that these compounds affect different stages of the life cycle of viruses: they block the first stage (attachment of the pathogen to the cell surface) of viral infection, prevent the spread of the virus and its ability to develop and acquire drug resistance, and also in some cases have a direct antiviral effect. PTs inhibit viral replication by blocking vital viral enzymes and preventing the release of viral particles from the cell. Other types of biological activities, i.e., anti-inflammatory, antioxidant, immunomodulatory and antitoxic, have become vitally important in case of late detection of the disease, its severe or complicated form, where the leading role in pathogenesis is played by reactive processes rather than by viral ones, complicated by bacterial infection. It should be noted that algal PPs affect vital processes that are common to severe viral inflammatory processes, irrespective the aetiology of the disease: the production of proinflammatory cytokines, cell migration to the inflammatory focus, etc. Therefore, algal PTs can be a basis for the development of drugs effectively acting on the innate immunity in various viral infections.

A combination of target technologies has shown numerous benefits in combating viral diseases. PTs from seaweed can be used in combination with officially approved drugs, which makes it possible to reduce the dose of these therapeutic agents and thereby reduce side effects. However, algae-derived PTs have been insufficiently studied to date, mainly in experiments. In this regard, it is necessary to extend research on the bioavailability of these compounds obtained from various seaweed species and the spectrum of their antiviral activities [99]. It should be determined which seaweed PPs have the strongest antiviral effect and which work best: whole seaweed, extracts enriched in PPs or PTs with a fixed structure. Another important question is do algae-derived PPs alter the composition and functioning of the intestinal microbiota? Furthermore, at last, can there be any undesirable effects caused by long-term use of different algal polyphenols at high doses?

Currently, the presence of complex polymer mixtures of their structural and conformational isomers in seaweed poses a serious challenge to researchers to characterise the composition of PTs, which is absolutely necessary for the development of pharmaceutical products. For this reason, only a selective structural characterisation of PTs is still possible [13]. It is also necessary to understand to what extent the results obtained in experiments with PP from seaweed in vitro can be extrapolated to their actual effects in a whole organism, and whether the very effective, but still poorly studied, compounds can be considered an alternative or supplement to the existing strategies for the treatment of viral diseases. Relevant material is still being accumulated; the analysis of this material may subsequently create conditions for the creation of medicinal antiviral drugs with a new mechanism of action, resistance to which in pathogens would not form.

In the current conditions of the ongoing pandemic, the results of studies on the targeted effects of algal polyphenols on coronaviruses seem very promising, although these studies have been carried out in vitro so far. This issue becomes especially relevant due to the lack of effective drugs, including synthetic ones, for the treatment of viral diseases such as the coronavirus infection. It is important that polyphenols (as has been established for polyphenols from terrestrial plants) do not cause side effects and are also not antagonistic to drugs used for viral infections [100].

Effective nutraceuticals, to be potentially developed on the basis of algal polyphenols, can also be used in the complex therapy of viral diseases. It is necessary to extend in vivo studies on laboratory animals, which subsequently will allow proceeding to clinical tests.

Thus, studies in recent years have shown that algal polyphenols are polyfunctional compounds and, therefore, they have a great potential as active ingredients for the creation of novel pharmaceutical substances with antiviral activity.

Author Contributions: N.N.B., concept, methodology, approval of the final review; B.G.A., idea and writing plan, approval of the final version, collection and analysis of literature, preparation of a draft manuscript; T.S.Z., writing a conclusion, proofreading the article; S.P.K., methodology, conceptualisation, validation; T.A.K., editing and validation of the article, collection and analysis of literature data; L.N.F., analysis and interpretation of data, preparation of the original layout; T.N.Z., collecting material, preparing the draft text; M.Y.S., preparing illustrations, preparation of the draft manuscript. All authors have read and agreed to the published version of the manuscript.

Funding: This work was supported by the RFBR grant 20-04-60212 "Integrated ecological and virological monitoring of coronaviruses in the ecosystems of the Far East".

Institutional Review Board Statement: Not applicable.

Informed Consent Statement: Not applicable.

Conflicts of Interest: The authors declare no conflict of interest.

References

1. Ryu, W.-S. Virus Life Cycle. *Mol. Virol. Hum. Pathog. Viruses* **2017**, *5*, 31–45.
2. Abdullah, A.A.; Abdullah, R.; Nazariah, Z.A.; Balakrishnan, K.N.; Abdullah, F.F.J.; Bala, J.A.; Mohd-Lila, M.-A. Cyclophilin A as a target in the treatment of cytomegalovirus infections. *Antivir. Chem. Chemother.* **2018**, *26*. [CrossRef]
3. Strasfeld, L.; Chou, S. Antiviral Drug Resistance: Mechanisms and Clinical Implications. *Infect. Dis. Clin. N. Am.* **2010**, *24*, 413–437. [CrossRef]
4. Irwin, K.K.; Renzette, N.; Kowalik, T.F.; Jensen, J.D. Antiviral drug resistance as an adaptive process. *Virus Evol.* **2016**, *2*, vew014. [CrossRef]
5. Hamed, I.; Özogul, F.; Özogul, Y.; Regenstein, J.M. Marine Bioactive Compounds and Their Health Benefits: A Review. *Compr. Rev. Food Sci. Food Saf.* **2015**, *14*, 446–465. [CrossRef]
6. Pedrosa, R.; Gaudêncio, S.P.; Vasconcelos, V. XVI International Symposium on Marine Natural Products l XI European Conference on Marine Natural Products. *Mar. Drugs* **2020**, *18*, 40. [CrossRef]
7. Moghaddam, J.A.; Dávila-Céspedes, A.; Kehraus, S.; Crüsemann, M.; Köse, M.; Müller, C.E.; König, G.M. Cyclopropane-Containing Fatty Acids from the Marine Bacterium Labrenzia sp. 011 with Antimicrobial and GPR84 Activity. *Mar. Drugs* **2018**, *16*, 369. [CrossRef]
8. Santhi, L.S.; Vssl, P.T.; Sy, N.; Radha Krishna, E. Bioactive Compounds from Marine Sponge Associates: Antibiotics from Bacillus sp. *Nat. Prod. Chem. Res.* **2017**, *5*, 4. [CrossRef]
9. Riccio, G.; Lauritano, C. Microalgae with Immunomodulatory Activities. *Mar. Drugs* **2019**, *18*, 2. [CrossRef]
10. Malve, H. Exploring the ocean for new drug developments: Marine pharmacology. *J. Pharm. Bioallied Sci.* **2016**, *8*, 83–91. [CrossRef] [PubMed]
11. Poole, J.; Diop, A.; Rainville, L.-C.; Barnabé, S. Bioextracting Polyphenols from the Brown Seaweed Ascophyllum nodosum from Québec's North Shore Coastline. *Ind. Biotechnol.* **2019**, *15*, 212–218. [CrossRef]
12. Gupta, S.; Abu-Ghannam, N. Recent developments in the application of seaweeds or seaweed extracts as a means for enhancing the safety and quality attributes of foods. *Innov. Food Sci. Emerg. Technol.* **2011**, *12*, 600–609. [CrossRef]
13. Имбс, Т.; Звягинцева, Т. ФЛОРОТАННИНЫ -ПОЛИФЕНОЛЬНЫЕ МЕТАБОЛИТЫ БУРЫХВОДОРОСЛЕЙ. Биология моря **2018**, *44*, 217–227. [CrossRef]
14. Heffernan, N.; Smyth, T.J.; Soler-Villa, A.; Fitzgerald, R.J.; Brunton, N.P. Phenolic content and antioxidant activity of fractions obtained from selected Irish macroalgae species (Laminaria digitate, Fucus serratus, Gracillaria gracilis and Codium fragile). *J. Appl. Phycol.* **2014**, *27*, 519–530. [CrossRef]
15. Shibata, T.; Kawaguchi, S.; Hama, Y.; Inagaki, M.; Yamaguchi, K.; Nakamura, T. Local and chemical distribution of phlorotannins in brown algae. *Environ. Biol. Fishes* **2004**, *16*, 291–296. [CrossRef]
16. Holdt, S.L.; Kraan, S. Bioactive compounds in seaweed: Functional food applications and legislation. *J. Appl. Phycol.* **2011**, *23*, 543–597. [CrossRef]
17. Sathya, M.; Kokilavani, R. Phitochemical screening and in vivo antioxidant activity of Saccharum spontaneous linn. *Int. J. Pharm. Sci. Rev. Res.* **2013**, *18*, 75–79.
18. Manandhar, S.; Luitel, S.; Dahal, R.K. In Vitro Antimicrobial Activity of Some Medicinal Plants against Human Pathogenic Bacteria. *J. Trop. Med.* **2019**, *2019*, 1895340. [CrossRef]
19. Singh, R.; Akhtar, N.; Haqqi, T.M. Green tea polyphenol epigallocatechi3-gallate: Inflammation and arthritis. *Life Sci.* **2010**, *86*, 907–918. [CrossRef] [PubMed]
20. Melanson, J.E.; MacKinnon, S.L. Characterization of Phlorotannins from Brown Algae by LC-HRMS. *Methods Mol. Biol.* **2015**, *1308*, 253–266. [CrossRef] [PubMed]
21. Montero, L.; Sánchez-Camargo, A.P.; García-Cañas, V.; Tanniou, A.; Stiger-Pouvreau, V.; Russo, M.; Rastrelli, L.; Cifuentes, A.; Herrero, M.; Ibáñez, E. Anti-proliferative activity and chemical characterization by comprehensive two-dimensional liquid chromatography coupled to mass spectrometry of phlorotannins from the brown macroalga Sargassum muticum collected on North-Atlantic coasts. *J. Chromatogr. A* **2016**, *1428*, 115–125. [CrossRef]
22. Swallah, M.S.; Fu, H.; Sun, H.; Affoh, R.; Yu, H. The Impact of Polyphenol on General Nutrient Metabolism in the Monogastric Gastrointestinal Tract. *J. Food Qual.* **2020**, *2020*, 1–12. [CrossRef]
23. Clifford, M.N. Diet-Derived Phenols in Plasma and Tissues and their Implications for Health. *Planta Med.* **2004**, *70*, 1103–1114. [CrossRef]
24. Lewandowska, U.; Szewczyk, K.; Hrabec, E.; Janecka, A.; Gorlach, S. Overview of Metabolism and Bioavailability Enhancement of Polyphenols. *J. Agric. Food Chem.* **2013**, *61*, 12183–12199. [CrossRef] [PubMed]
25. Ragan, M.A.; Glombitza, K.W. Phlorotannins, brown algal polyphenols. *Prog. Phycol. Res.* **1986**, *4*, 129–241.
26. Pádua, D.; Rocha, E.; Gargiulo, D.; Ramos, A. Bioactive compounds from brown seaweeds: Phloroglucinol, fucoxanthin and fucoidan as promising therapeutic agents against breast cancer. *Phytochem. Lett.* **2015**, *14*, 91–98. [CrossRef]
27. Mannino, A.M.; Micheli, C. Ecological Function of Phenolic Compounds from Mediterranean Fucoid Algae and Seagrasses: An Overview on the Genus *Cystoseira sensu lato* and *Posidonia oceanica* (L.) Delile. *J. Mar. Sci. Eng.* **2020**, *8*, 19. [CrossRef]
28. Li, A.-N.; Li, S.; Zhang, Y.-J.; Xu, X.-R.; Chen, Y.-M.; Li, H.-B. Resources and Biological Activities of Natural Polyphenols. *Nutrients* **2014**, *6*, 6020–6047. [CrossRef] [PubMed]

29. Rengasamy, K.R.; Aderogba, M.A.; Amoo, S.O.; Stirk, W.A.; Van Staden, J. Potential antiradical and alpha-glucosidase inhibitors from Ecklonia maxima (Osbeck) Papenfuss. *Food Chem.* **2013**, *141*, 1412–1415. [CrossRef] [PubMed]
30. Kim, A.-R.; Shin, T.-S.; Lee, M.-S.; Park, J.-Y.; Park, K.-E.; Yoon, N.-Y.; Kim, J.-S.; Choi, J.-S.; Jang, B.-C.; Byun, D.-S.; et al. Isolation and Identification of Phlorotannins from Ecklonia stolonifera with Antioxidant and Anti-inflammatory Properties. *J. Agric. Food Chem.* **2009**, *57*, 3483–3489. [CrossRef]
31. Li, Y.; Lee, S.-H.; Le, Q.-T.; Kim, M.-M.; Kim, S.-K. Anti-allergic Effects of Phlorotannins on Histamine Release via Binding Inhibition between IgE and FcεRI. *J. Agric. Food Chem.* **2008**, *56*, 12073–12080. [CrossRef] [PubMed]
32. Ahn, M.-J.; Yoon, K.-D.; Min, S.-Y.; Lee, J.S.; Kim, J.H.; Kim, T.G.; Kim, S.H.; Kim, N.-G.; Huh, H.; Kim, J. Inhibition of HIV-1 Reverse Transcriptase and Protease by Phlorotannins from the Brown Alga Ecklonia cava. *Biol. Pharm. Bull.* **2004**, *27*, 544–547. [CrossRef] [PubMed]
33. Catarino, M.D.; Silva, A.M.S.; Cardoso, S.M. Fucaceae: A Source of Bioactive Phlorotannins. *Int. J. Mol. Sci.* **2017**, *18*, 1327. [CrossRef]
34. Lee, S.-H.; Jeon, Y.-J. Anti-diabetic effects of brown algae derived phlorotannins, marine polyphenols through diverse mechanisms. *Fitoterapia* **2013**, *86*, 129–136. [CrossRef]
35. Garcia-Vaquero, M.; Ummat, V.; Tiwari, B.; Rajauria, G. Exploring Ultrasound, Microwave and Ultrasound–Microwave Assisted Extraction Technologies to Increase the Extraction of Bioactive Compounds and Antioxidants from Brown Macroalgae. *Mar. Drugs* **2020**, *18*, 172. [CrossRef]
36. Koivikko, R.; Eranen, J.K.; Loponen, J.; Jormalainen, Y. Variation of phlorotannins among three populations of Fucus vesic-ulosus as revealed by HPLC and colorimetric quantification. *J. Chem. Ecol.* **2008**, *34*, 57–64. [CrossRef] [PubMed]
37. Firquet, S.; Beaujard, S.; Lobert, P.-E.; Sané, F.; Caloone, D.; Izard, D.; Hober, D. Survival of Enveloped and Non-Enveloped Viruses on Inanimate Surfaces. *Microbes Environ.* **2015**, *30*, 140–144. [CrossRef] [PubMed]
38. Wink, M. Modes of Action of Herbal Medicines and Plant Secondary Metabolites. *Medicines* **2015**, *2*, 251–286. [CrossRef] [PubMed]
39. Wink, M. Potential of DNA intercalating alcaloids and other plant secondary metabolites against SARS-CoV-2 causing COVID-19. *Diversity* **2020**, *12*, 175. [CrossRef]
40. Venkatesan, J.; Keekan, K.K.; Anil, S.; Bhatnagar, I.; Kim, S.-K. Phlorotannins. *Encycl. Food Chem.* **2019**, *27*, 515–527. [CrossRef]
41. Yang, H.-K.; Jung, M.-H.; Avunje, S.; Nikapitiya, C.; Kang, S.Y.; Ryu, Y.B.; Lee, W.S.; Jung, S.-J. Efficacy of algal Ecklonia cava extract against viral hemorrhagic septicemia virus (VHSV). *Fish Shellfish. Immunol.* **2018**, *72*, 273–281. [CrossRef]
42. Kwon, H.-J.; Ryu, Y.B.; Kim, Y.-M.; Song, N.; Kim, C.Y.; Rho, M.-C.; Jeong, J.-H.; Cho, K.-O.; Lee, W.S.; Park, S.-J. In vitro antiviral activity of phlorotannins isolated from Ecklonia cava against porcine epidemic diarrhea coronavirus infection and hemagglutination. *Bioorgan. Med. Chem.* **2013**, *21*, 4706–4713. [CrossRef]
43. Ueda, K.; Kawabata, R.; Irie, T.; Nakai, Y.; Tohya, Y.; Sakaguchi, T. Inactivation of Pathogenic Viruses by Plant-Derived Tannins: Strong Effects of Extracts from Persimmon (Diospyros kaki) on a Broad Range of Viruses. *PLOS ONE* **2013**, *8*, e55343. [CrossRef] [PubMed]
44. Cho, H.M.; Doan, T.P.; Ha, T.K.Q.; Kim, H.W.; Lee, B.W.; Pham, H.T.T.; Cho, T.O.; Oh, W.K. Dereplication by High-Performance Liquid Chromatography (HPLC) with Quadrupole-Time-of-Flight Mass Spectroscopy (qTOF-MS) and Antiviral Activities of Phlorotannins from Ecklonia cava. *Mar. Drugs* **2019**, *17*, 149. [CrossRef] [PubMed]
45. Khokhlova, N.I.; Kapustin, D.V.; Krasnova, E.I.; Izvekova, I.Y.I. NOROVIRUS INFECTION (SYSTEMATIC REVIEW). *J. Infectol.* **2018**, *10*, 5–14. [CrossRef]
46. La Rosa, G.; Muscillo, M. Molecular detection of viruses in water and sewage. In *Viruses in Food and Water*; Elsevier: Amsterdam, The Netherlands, 2013; pp. 97–125.
47. Atmar, R.L. Noroviruses: State of the Art. *Food Environ. Virol.* **2010**, *2*, 117–126. [CrossRef]
48. Choi, Y.; Kim, E.; Moon, S.; Choi, J.-D.; Lee, M.-S.; Kim, Y.-M. Phaeophyta Extracts Exhibit Antiviral Activity against Feline Calicivirus. *Fish. Aquat. Sci.* **2014**, *17*, 155–158. [CrossRef]
49. Eom, S.H.; Moon, S.Y.; Lee, D.S.; Kim, H.J.; Park, K.; Lee, E.W.; Kim, T.H.; Chung, Y.H.; Lee, M.S.; Kim, Y.M. In vitro antiviral activity of dieckol and phlorofucofuroecko-A isolated from edible brown alga Eisenia bicyclis against murine norovirus. *Algae* **2015**, *30*, 241–246. [CrossRef]
50. Bailey-Elkin, B.A.; Knaap, R.C.; Kikkert, M.; Mark, B.L. Structure and Function of Viral Deubiquitinating Enzymes. *J. Mol. Biol.* **2017**, *429*, 3441–3470. [CrossRef] [PubMed]
51. Lee, T.-W.; Cherney, M.M.; Liu, J.; James, K.E.; Powers, J.C.; Eltis, L.D.; James, M.N. Crystal Structures Reveal an Induced-fit Binding of a Substrate-like Aza-peptide Epoxide to SARS Coronavirus Main Peptidase. *J. Mol. Biol.* **2007**, *366*, 916–932. [CrossRef] [PubMed]
52. Xu, Z.; Peng, C.; Shi, Y.; Zhu, Z.; Mu, K.; Wang, X.; Zhu, W. Nelfinavir was predicted to be a potential inhibitor of 2019-nCov main protease by an inte-grative approach combining homology modelling, molecular docking and binding free energy calculation. *BioRxiv* **2020**. [CrossRef]
53. Rathnayake, A.D.; Zheng, J.; Kim, Y.; Perera, K.D.; Mackin, S.; Meyerholz, D.K.; Kashipathy, M.M.; Battaile, K.P.; Lovell, S.; Perlman, S.; et al. 3C-like protease inhibitors block coronavirus replication in vitro and improve survival in MERS-CoV–infected mice. *Sci. Transl. Med.* **2020**, *12*, eabc5332. [CrossRef]
54. Skvortsov, V.; Druzhilovskiy, D.; Veselovsky, A. Potential inhibitors of protease 3CLpro virus COVID-19: Drug reposition. *Biomed. Chem. Res. Methods* **2020**, *3*, e00124. [CrossRef]

55. Ho, T.-Y.; Wu, S.-L.; Chen, J.-C.; Li, C.-C.; Hsiang, C.-Y. Emodin blocks the SARS coronavirus spike protein and angiotensin-converting enzyme 2 interaction. *Antivir. Res.* **2007**, *74*, 92–101. [CrossRef] [PubMed]
56. Hulswit, R.J.; De Haan, C.A.; Bosch, B.J. Coronavirus Spike Protein and Tropism Changes. *Adv. Virus Res.* **2016**, *96*, 29–57. [CrossRef] [PubMed]
57. Park, J.-Y.; Yuk, H.J.; Ryu, H.W.; Lim, S.H.; Kim, K.S.; Park, K.H.; Ryu, Y.B.; Lee, W.S. Evaluation of polyphenols from Broussonetia papyrifera as coronavirus protease inhibitors. *J. Enzym. Inhib. Med. Chem.* **2017**, *32*, 504–512. [CrossRef] [PubMed]
58. Piccolella, S.; Crescente, G.; Faramarzi, S.; Formato, M.; Pecoraro, M.T.; Pacifico, S. Polyphenols vs. Coronaviruses: How Far Has Research Moved Forward? *Molecules* **2020**, *25*, 4103. [CrossRef] [PubMed]
59. Nicholls, J.M.; Chan, R.W.; Russell, R.J.; Air, G.M.; Peiris, J.M. Evolving complexities of influenza virus and its receptors. *Trends Microbiol.* **2008**, *16*, 149–157. [CrossRef] [PubMed]
60. Park, J.-Y.; Kim, J.H.; Kwon, J.M.; Kwon, H.-J.; Jeong, H.J.; Kim, Y.M.; Kim, D.; Lee, W.S.; Ryu, Y.B. Dieckol, a SARS-CoV 3CLpro inhibitor, isolated from the edible brown algae Ecklonia cava. *Bioorgan. Med. Chem.* **2013**, *21*, 3730–3737. [CrossRef] [PubMed]
61. Singh, S.B.; Liu, W.; Li, X.; Chen, T.; Shafiee, A.; Card, D.; Abruzzo, G.; Flattery, A.; Gill, C.; Thompson, J.R.; et al. Antifungal Spectrum, In Vivo Efficacy, and Structure–Activity Relationship of Ilicicolin H. *ACS Med. Chem. Lett.* **2012**, *3*, 814–817. [CrossRef] [PubMed]
62. Singh, S.B.; Liu, W.; Li, X.; Chen, T.; Shafiee, A.; Dreikorn, S.; Hornak, V.; Meinz, M.; Onishi, J.C. Structure–activity relationship of cytochrome bc1 reductase inhibitor broad spectrum antifungal ilicicolin H. *Bioorgan. Med. Chem. Lett.* **2013**, *23*, 3018–3022. [CrossRef]
63. Ryu, Y.B.; Jeong, H.J.; Yoon, S.Y.; Park, J.-Y.; Kim, Y.M.; Park, S.-J.; Rho, M.-C.; Kim, S.-J.; Lee, W.S. Influenza Virus Neuraminidase Inhibitory Activity of Phlorotannins from the Edible Brown AlgaEcklonia cava. *J. Agric. Food Chem.* **2011**, *59*, 6467–6473. [CrossRef]
64. Vo, T.-S.; Kim, S.-K. Potential Anti-HIV Agents from Marine Resources: An Overview. *Mar. Drugs* **2010**, *8*, 2871–2892. [CrossRef] [PubMed]
65. Ahn, M.-J.; Yoon, K.-D.; Kim, C.Y.; Shin, C.-G.; Kim, J.H.; Kim, J. Inhibitory activity on HIV-1 reverse transcriptase and integrase of a carmalol derivative from a brown Alga, Ishige okamurae. *Phytotherapy Res.* **2006**, *20*, 711–713. [CrossRef]
66. Artan, M.; Li, Y.; Karadeniz, F.; Lee, S.-H.; Kim, M.-M.; Kim, S.-K. Anti-HIV-1 activity of phloroglucinol derivative, 6,6′-bieckol, from Ecklonia cava. *Bioorganic. Med. Chem.* **2008**, *16*, 7921–7926. [CrossRef] [PubMed]
67. Karadeniz, F.; Kang, K.-H.; Park, J.W.; Park, S.-J.; Kim, S.-K. Anti-HIV-1 activity of phlorotannin derivative 8,4‴-dieckol from Korean brown algaEcklonia cava. *Biosci. Biotechnol. Biochem.* **2014**, *78*, 1151–1158. [CrossRef]
68. Benarba, B.; Pandiella, A. Medicinal Plants as Sources of Active Molecules Against COVID-19. *Front. Pharmacol.* **2020**, *11*, 1189. [CrossRef] [PubMed]
69. De Mello, C.P.P.; Drusano, G.L.; Rodriquez, J.L.; Kaushik, A.; Brown, A.N. Antiviral Effects of Clinically-Relevant Interferon-α and Ribavirin Regimens against Dengue Virus in the Hollow Fiber Infection Model (HFIM). *Viruses* **2018**, *10*, 317. [CrossRef] [PubMed]
70. Morán-Santibañez, K.; Peña-Hernández, M.A.; Cruz-Suárez, L.E.; Ricque-Marie, D.; Skouta, R.; Vasquez, A.H.; Rodríguez-Padilla, C.; Trejo-Avila, L.M. Virucidal and Synergistic Activity of Polyphenol-Rich Extracts of Seaweeds against Measles Virus. *Viruses* **2018**, *10*, 465. [CrossRef]
71. Xi, C.; Zhang, Y.; Marrs, C.F.; Ye, W.; Simon, C.; Foxman, B.; Nriagu, J. Prevalence of Antibiotic Resistance in Drinking Water Treatment and Distribution Systems. *Appl. Environ. Microbiol.* **2009**, *75*, 5714–5718. [CrossRef] [PubMed]
72. Valyi-Nagy, T.; Dermody, T.S. Role of oxidative damage in the pathogenesis of viral infections of the nervous system. *Histol. Histopathol.* **2005**, *20*, 957–967.
73. Fedoreyev, S.A.; Krylova, N.V.; Mishchenko, N.P.; Vasileva, E.A.; Pislyagin, E.A.; Iunikhina, O.V.; Lavrov, V.F.; Svitich, O.A.; Ebralidze, L.K.; Leonova, G.N. Antiviral and Antioxidant Properties of Echinochrome A. *Mar. Drugs* **2018**, *16*, 509. [CrossRef] [PubMed]
74. Bhattacharya, S. Reactive Oxygen Species and Cellular Defense System. In *Free Radicals in Human Health and Disease*; Rani, V., Yadav, U.C.S., Eds.; Springer: New Delhi, India, 2015; pp. 17–29.
75. Bakunina, N.; Pariante, C.M.; Zunszain, P.A. Immune mechanisms linked to depression via oxidative stress and neuropro-gression. *Immunology* **2015**, *144*, 365–373. [CrossRef]
76. Sansone, C.; Brunet, C.; Noonan, D.M.; Albini, A. Marine Algal Antioxidants as Potential Vectors for Controlling Viral Diseases. *Antioxidants* **2020**, *9*, 392. [CrossRef]
77. Gullberg, R.C.; Steel, J.J.; Moon, S.L.; Soltani, E.; Geiss, B.J. Oxidative stress influences positive strand RNA virus genome synthesis and capping. *Virology* **2015**, *475*, 219–229. [CrossRef] [PubMed]
78. Sebastiano, M.; Chastel, O.; De Thoisy, B.; Eens, M.; Costantini, D. Oxidative stress favours herpes virus infection in vertebrates: A meta-analysis. *Curr. Zoöl.* **2016**, *62*, 325–332. [CrossRef]
79. Kavouras, J.H.; Prandovszky, E.; Valyi-Nagy, K.; Kovacs, S.K.; Tiwari, V.; Kovács, M.; Shukla, D.; Valyi-Nagy, T. Herpes simplex virus type 1 infection induces oxidative stress and the release of bioactive lipid peroxidation by-products in mouse P19N neural cell cultures. *J. NeuroVirol.* **2007**, *13*, 416–425. [CrossRef]
80. Chen, X.; Kamranvar, S.A.; Masucci, M.G. Oxidative stress enables Epstein–Barr virus-induced B-cell transformation by posttran-scriptional regulation of viral and cellular growth-promoting factors. *Oncogene* **2016**, *35*, 3807–3816. [CrossRef] [PubMed]

81. Firuzi, O.; Miri, R.; Tavakkoli, M.; Saso, L. Antioxidant Therapy: Current Status and Future Prospects. *Curr. Med. Chem.* **2011**, *18*, 3871–3888. [CrossRef]
82. Fassina, G.; Buffa, A.; Benelli, R.; Varnier, O.E.; Noonan, D.M.; Albini, A. Polyphenolic antioxidant (–)-epigallocatechin-3-gallate from green tea as a candidate anti-HIV agent. *AIDS* **2002**, *16*, 939–941. [CrossRef] [PubMed]
83. Mathew, D.; Hsu, W.-L. Antiviral potential of curcumin. *J. Funct. Foods* **2018**, *40*, 692–699. [CrossRef]
84. Di Sotto, A.; Checconi, P.; Celestino, I.; Locatelli, M.; Carissimi, S.; De Angelis, M.; Rossi, V.; Limongi, D.; Toniolo, C.; Martinoli, L.; et al. Antiviral and Antioxidant Activity of a Hydroalcoholic Extract from *Humulus lupulus* L. *Oxidative Med. Cell. Longev.* **2018**, *2018*, 5919237. [CrossRef] [PubMed]
85. Reshi, M.L.; Su, Y.-C.; Hong, J.-R. RNA Viruses: ROS-Mediated Cell Death. *Int. J. Cell Biol.* **2014**, *2014*, 467452. [CrossRef]
86. Dasuri, K.; Zhang, L.; Keller, J.N. Oxidative stress, neurodegeneration, and the balance of protein degradation and protein synthesis. *Free. Radic. Biol. Med.* **2013**, *62*, 170–185. [CrossRef]
87. Palus, M.; Bílý, T.; Elsterová, J.; Langhansová, H.; Salát, J.; Vancová, M.; Růžek, D. Infection and injury of human astrocytes by tick-borne encephalitis virus. *J. Gen. Virol.* **2014**, *95*, 2411–2426. [CrossRef] [PubMed]
88. Krylova, N.V.; Popov, A.M.; Leonova, G.N. Antioxidants as Potential Antiviral Drugs for Flavivirus Infections. *Antibiot. Chemother.* **2016**, *61*, 25–30. (In Russia)
89. Popov, A.M.; Artyukov, A.A.; Krivoshapko, O.N.; Krylova, N.V.; Leonova, G.N.; Kozlovskaja, E.P. An Agent with Antioxidant, Cardioprotective, Antidiabetic, Anti-Inflammatory, Hepatoprotective, Anti-Tumor and Antiviral Effects. RF Patent C1 2432959, 2011. (In Russia)
90. Krylova, N.V.; Popov, A.M.; Leonova, G.N.; Artiukov, A.A.; Maĭstrovskaia, O.S. Study of the activity of the drug Luromarin in vitro against tick-borne encephalitis virus. *Antibiot. Chemother.* **2010**, *55*, 17–19.
91. Krylova, N.V.; Popov, A.M.; Leonova, G.N.; Artiukov, A.A.; Maĭstrovskaia, O.S. Comparative study of the antiviral activity of luteolin and luteolin 7,3'-disulfate. *Antibiot. Chemother.* **2011**, *56*, 7–10.
92. Lee, S.H.; Eom, S.H.; Yoon, N.Y.; Kim, M.K.; Li, Y.X.; Ha, S.K.; Kim, S.K. Fucofuroeckol-A from Eisenia bicyclis inhibits inflammation in lipopolysaccha-ride-induced mouse macrophages via downregulation of the MAPK/NF-kB signaling pathway. *J. Chem.* **2016**, 6509212. (In Russia)
93. Montero-Lobato, Z.; Vázquez, M.; Navarro, F.; Fuentes, J.L.; Bermejo, E.; Garbayo, I.; Vílchez, C.; Cuaresma, M. Chemically-Induced Production of Anti-Inflammatory Molecules in Microalgae. *Mar. Drugs* **2018**, *16*, 478. [CrossRef]
94. Sheikh, F.; Dickensheets, H.; Gamero, A.M.; Vogel, S.N.; Donnelly, R.P. An essential role for IFN-β in the induction of IFN-stimulated gene expression by LPS in macrophages. *J. Leukoc. Biol.* **2014**, *96*, 591–600. [CrossRef]
95. Yang, Y.-I.; Jung, S.-H.; Lee, K.-T.; Choi, J.-H. 8,8'-Bieckol, isolated from edible brown algae, exerts its anti-inflammatory effects through inhibition of NF-κB signaling and ROS production in LPS-stimulated macrophages. *Int. Immunopharmacol.* **2014**, *23*, 460–468. [CrossRef] [PubMed]
96. Li, S.; Liu, J.; Zhang, M.; Chen, Y.; Zhu, T.; Wang, J. Protective Effect of Eckol against Acute Hepatic Injury Induced by Carbon Tetrachloride in Mice. *Mar. Drugs* **2018**, *16*, 300. [CrossRef] [PubMed]
97. Zhang, M.-Y.; Guo, J.; Hu, X.-M.; Zhao, S.-Q.; Li, S.-L.; Wang, J. An in vivo anti-tumor effect of eckol from marine brown algae by improving the immune response. *Food Funct.* **2019**, *10*, 4361–4371. [CrossRef] [PubMed]
98. Zhen, A.X.; Hyun, Y.J.; Piao, M.J.; Fernando, P.D.S.M.; Kang, K.A.; Ahn, M.J.; Yi, J.M.; Kang, H.K.; Koh, Y.S.; Lee, N.H.; et al. Eckol Inhibits Particulate Matter 2.5-Induced Skin Keratinocyte Damage via MAPK Signaling Pathway. *Mar. Drugs* **2019**, *17*, 444. [CrossRef]
99. Kroon, P.A.; Clifford, M.N.; Crozier, A.; Day, A.J.; Donovan, J.L.; Manach, C.; Williamson, G. How should we assess the effects of exposure to dietary polyphenols in vitro? *Am. J. Clin. Nutr.* **2004**, *80*, 15–21. [CrossRef]
100. Landete, J.M. Updated Knowledge about Polyphenols: Functions, Bioavailability, Metabolism, and Health. *Crit. Rev. Food Sci. Nutr.* **2012**, *52*, 936–948. [CrossRef] [PubMed]
101. Manach, C.; Williamson, G.; Morand, C.; Scalbert, A.; Rémésy, C. Bioavailability and bioefficacy of polyphenols in humans. I. Review of 97 bioavailability studies. *Am. J. Clin. Nutr.* **2005**, *81*, 230S–242S. [CrossRef]
102. Williamson, G.; Manach, C. Bioavailability and bioefficacy of polyphenols in humans. II. Review of 93 intervention studies. *Am. J. Clin. Nutr.* **2005**, *81*, 243S–255S. [CrossRef] [PubMed]
103. Kelly, G.S. Quercetin Monograph. *Altern. Med. Rev.* **2011**, *16*, 172–194.
104. Mehrbod, P.; Hudy, D.; Shyntum, D.; Markowski, J.; Łos, M.J.; Ghavami, S. Quercetin as a Natural Therapeutic Candidate for the Treatment of Influenza Virus. *Biomolecules* **2020**, *11*, 10. [CrossRef]
105. Choi, H.J.; Song, J.H.; Kwon, D.H. Quercetin 3-rhamnoside Exerts Antiinfluenza A Virus Activity in Mice. *Phytother. Res.* **2011**, *26*, 462–464. [CrossRef] [PubMed]
106. Makarova, M.N. Bioavailability and metabolism of flavonoids. *Vopr. Pitan.* **2011**, *80*, 33–40.
107. Msc, T.A.N.R.; Lakshmi, A.N.V.; Anand, T.; Rao, L.V.; Sharma, G. Protective effects of quercetin during influenza virus-induced oxidative stress. *Asia Pac. J. Clin. Nutr.* **2000**, *9*, 314–317. [CrossRef]
108. Savov, V.M.; Galabov, A.S.; Tantcheva, L.P.; Mileva, M.M.; Pavlova, E.L.; Stoeva, E.S.; Braykova, A.A. Effects of rutin and quercetin on monooxygenase activities in experimental influenza virus infection. *Exp. Toxicol. Pathol.* **2006**, *58*, 59–64. [CrossRef] [PubMed]
109. Davis, J.M.; Murphy, E.A.; McClellan, J.L.; Carmichael, M.D.; Gangemi, J.D. Quercetin reduces susceptibility to influenza infection following stressful exercise. *Am. J. Physiol. Integr. Comp. Physiol.* **2008**, *295*, R505–R509. [CrossRef]

110. Ganesan, S.; Faris, A.N.; Comstock, A.T.; Wang, Q.; Nanua, S.; Hershenson, M.B.; Sajjan, U.S. Quercetin inhibits rhinovirus replication in vitro and in vivo. *Antivir. Res.* **2012**, *94*, 258–271. [CrossRef]
111. Newcomb, D.C.; Sajjan, U.S.; Nagarkar, D.R.; Wang, Q.; Nanua, S.; Zhou, Y.; McHenry, C.L.; Hennrick, K.T.; Tsai, W.C.; Bentley, J.K.; et al. Human Rhinovirus 1B Exposure Induces Phosphatidylinositol 3-Kinase–dependent Airway Inflammation in Mice. *Am. J. Respir. Crit. Care Med.* **2008**, *177*, 1111–1121. [CrossRef] [PubMed]
112. Sajjan, U.; Ganesan, S.; Comstock, A.T.; Shim, J.; Wang, Q.; Nagarkar, D.R.; Zhao, Y.; Goldsmith, A.M.; Sonstein, J.; Linn, M.J.; et al. Elastase- and LPS-exposed mice display altered responses to rhinovirus infection. *Am. J. Physiol. Cell. Mol. Physiol.* **2009**, *297*, L931–L944. [CrossRef] [PubMed]
113. Galochkina, A.V.; Anikin, V.B.; Babkin, V.A.; Ostrouhova, L.A.; Zarubaev, V.V. Virus-inhibiting activity of dihydroquercetin, a flavonoid from Larix sibirica, against coxsackievirus B4 in a model of viral pancreatitis. *Arch. Virol.* **2016**, *161*, 929–938. [CrossRef] [PubMed]
114. Qiu, X.; Kroeker, A.; He, S.; Kozak, R.; Audet, J.; Mbikay, M.; Chrétien, M. Prophylactic Efficacy of Quercetin 3-β-O-d-Glucoside against Ebola Virus Infection. *Antimicrob. Agents Chemother.* **2016**, *60*, 5182–5188. [CrossRef] [PubMed]
115. Kashyap, D.; Garg, V.K.; Tuli, H.S.; Yerer, M.B.; Sak, K.; Sharma, A.K.; Kumar, M.; Aggarwal, V.; Sandhu, S.S. Fisetin and Quercetin: Promising Flavonoids with Chemopreventive Potential. *Biomolecules* **2019**, *9*, 174. [CrossRef]
116. Nagai, T.; Suzuki, Y.; Tomimori, T.; Yamada, H. Antiviral Activity of Plant Flavonoid, 5,7,4′-Trihydroxy-8-methoxyflavone, from the Roots of Scutellaria baicalensis against Influenza A (H3N2) and B Viruses. *Biol. Pharm. Bull.* **1995**, *18*, 295–299. [CrossRef]
117. Ding, Y.; Dou, J.; Teng, Z.; Yu, J.; Wang, T.; Lu, N.; Wang, H.; Zhou, C. Antiviral activity of baicalin against influenza A (H1N1/H3N2) virus in cell culture and in mice and its inhibition of neuraminidase. *Arch. Virol.* **2014**, *159*, 3269–3278. [CrossRef] [PubMed]
118. Chu, M.; Xu, L.; Zhang, M.-B.; Chu, Z.-Y.; Wang, Y.-D. Role of Baicalin in Anti-Influenza Virus A as a Potent Inducer of IFN-Gamma. *BioMed Res. Int.* **2015**, *2015*, 263630. [CrossRef] [PubMed]
119. Dou, J.; Chen, L.; Xu, G.; Zhang, L.; Zhou, H.; Wang, H.; Su, Z.; Ke, M.; Guo, Q.; Zhou, C. Effects of baicalein on Sendai virus in vivo are linked to serum baicalin and its inhibition of hemagglutinin-neuraminidase. *Arch. Virol.* **2011**, *156*, 793–801. [CrossRef] [PubMed]
120. Zang, N.; Xie, X.; Deng, Y.; Wu, S.; Wang, L.; Peng, C.; Li, S.; Ni, K.; Luo, Y.; Liu, E. Resveratrol-Mediated Gamma Interferon Reduction Prevents Airway Inflammation and Airway Hyperresponsiveness in Respiratory Syncytial Virus-Infected Immunocompromised Mice. *J. Virol.* **2011**, *85*, 13061–13068. [CrossRef]
121. Huang, H.; Liao, D.; Zhou, G.; Zhu, Z.; Cui, Y.; Pu, R. Antiviral activities of resveratrol against rotavirus in vitro and in vivo. *Phytomedicine* **2020**, *77*, 153230. [CrossRef] [PubMed]
122. Matsumoto, K.; Yamada, H.; Takuma, N.; Niino, H.; Sagesaka, Y.M. Effects of Green Tea Catechins and Theanine on Preventing Influenza Infection among Healthcare Workers: A Randomized Controlled Trial. *BMC Complement. Altern. Med.* **2011**, *11*, 15. [CrossRef] [PubMed]
123. O'Shea, D.; Law, J.; Egli, A.; Douglas, D.; Lund, G.; Forester, S.; Lambert, J.; Law, M.; Burton, D.R.; Tyrrell, D.L.J.; et al. Prevention of hepatitis C virus infection using a broad cross-neutralizing monoclonal antibody (AR4A) and epigallocatechin gallate. *Liver Transplant.* **2015**, *22*, 324–332. [CrossRef] [PubMed]

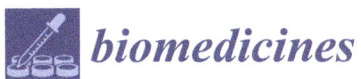

Article

Caffeic Acid, One of the Major Phenolic Acids of the Medicinal Plant *Antirhea borbonica*, Reduces Renal Tubulointerstitial Fibrosis

Bryan Veeren [1], Matthieu Bringart [1], Chloe Turpin [1], Philippe Rondeau [1], Cynthia Planesse [1], Imade Ait-Arsa [2], Fanny Gimié [2], Claude Marodon [3], Olivier Meilhac [1], Marie-Paule Gonthier [1], Nicolas Diotel [1] and Jean-Loup Bascands [1,*]

[1] Diabète Athérothrombose Thérapies Réunion Océan Indien, INSERM, UMR 1188, Université de La Réunion, 2 Rue Maxime Rivière, 97490 Sainte-Clotilde, France; bryan.veeren@univ-reunion.fr (B.V.); matthieu.bringart@inserm.fr (M.B.); chloe.turpin@univ-reunion.fr (C.T.); philippe.rondeau@univ-reunion.fr (P.R.); cynthia.planesse@univ-reunion.fr (C.P.); olivier.meilhac@inserm.fr (O.M.); marie-paule.gonthier@univ-reunion.fr (M.-P.G.); nicolas.diotel@univ-reunion.fr (N.D.)

[2] Groupe d'Intérêt Public, Cyclotron Réunion Océan Indien, 2 Rue Maxime Rivière, 97490 Réunion, France; i.aitarsa@cyroi.fr (I.A.-A.); f.gimie@cyroi.fr (F.G.)

[3] Aplamedon Réunion, CYROI-Parc Technor—2, Rue Maxime Rivière, 97490 Réunion, France; claude.marodon@aplamedom.com

* Correspondence: jean-loup.bascands@inserm.fr; Tel.: +262-262-938806

Abstract: The renal fibrotic process is characterized by a chronic inflammatory state and oxidative stress. *Antirhea borbonica* (*A. borbonica*) is a French medicinal plant found in Reunion Island and known for its antioxidant and anti-inflammatory activities mostly related to its high polyphenols content. We investigated whether oral administration of polyphenol-rich extract from *A. borbonica* could exert in vivo a curative anti-renal fibrosis effect. To this aim, three days after unilateral ureteral obstruction (UUO), mice were daily orally treated either with a non-toxic dose of polyphenol-rich extract from *A. borbonica* or with caffeic acid (CA) for 5 days. The polyphenol-rich extract from *A. borbonica*, as well as CA, the predominant phenolic acid of this medicinal plant, exerted a nephroprotective effect through the reduction in the three phases of the fibrotic process: (i) macrophage infiltration, (ii) myofibroblast appearance and (iii) extracellular matrix accumulation. These effects were associated with the mRNA down-regulation of *Tgf-β*, *Tnf-α*, *Mcp1* and *NfkB*, as well as the upregulation of *Nrf2*. Importantly, we observed an increased antioxidant enzyme activity for GPX and Cu/ZnSOD. Last but not least, desorption electrospray ionization-high resolution/mass spectrometry (DESI-HR/MS) imaging allowed us to visualize, for the first time, CA in the kidney tissue. The present study demonstrates that polyphenol-rich extract from *A. borbonica* significantly improves, in a curative way, renal tubulointerstitial fibrosis progression in the UUO mouse model.

Keywords: *Antirhea borbonica*; kidney fibrosis; polyphenols; caffeic acid; antioxidant enzymes; DESI-imaging

1. Introduction

A common deleterious consequence of most chronic kidney diseases (CKD) is the interstitial accumulation of extracellular matrix leading to tubulointerstitial fibrosis, which is closely correlated with the loss of renal function [1–4]. The process of renal fibrosis can be seen as an ongoing wound-healing process maintained by a chronic inflammatory reaction [5,6]. Halting renal fibrosis progression appears as a relevant therapeutic strategy to at least delay CKD progression. Although significant progress in the understanding of the molecular mechanisms occurring during fibrosis has been made [6], specific antifibrotic drugs and/or treatments are still clearly lacking. To the best of our knowledge the only drugs used in clinic to slow down the progression of CKD are angiotensin-converting

---

Citation: Veeren, B.; Bringart, M.; Turpin, C.; Rondeau, P.; Planesse, C.; Ait-Arsa, I.; Gimié, F.; Marodon, C.; Meilhac, O.; Gonthier, M.-P.; et al. Caffeic Acid, One of the Major Phenolic Acids of the Medicinal Plant *Antirhea borbonica*, Reduces Renal Tubulointerstitial Fibrosis. *Biomedicines* 2021, 9, 358. https://doi.org/10.3390/biomedicines9040358

Academic Editors: Mario Dell'Agli and Enrico Sangiovanni

Received: 3 March 2021
Accepted: 27 March 2021
Published: 30 March 2021

Publisher's Note: MDPI stays neutral with regard to jurisdictional claims in published maps and institutional affiliations.

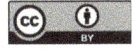

Copyright: © 2021 by the authors. Licensee MDPI, Basel, Switzerland. This article is an open access article distributed under the terms and conditions of the Creative Commons Attribution (CC BY) license (https://creativecommons.org/licenses/by/4.0/).

enzyme inhibitors and angiotensin type I receptor blockers [7–9]. Diabetic kidney disease remains the main cause of CKD, leading to end-stage kidney disease in both type 1 and type 2 diabetes [10]. Recently, sodium–glucose linked transporter-2 (SGLT2) inhibitors appeared to be the most promising nephroprotective drugs in diabetic kidney disease [11,12]; however, an antifibrotic effect has only been evidenced in animal studies [13]. There is thus a need and ample space to develop new therapeutic approaches targeting tubulointerstitial fibrosis in the kidney for combatting these pathological processes [14].

Chronic infiltration of immune cells in renal tissue, as well as chronic hypoxia and oxidative stress, are clearly involved in the initiation and progression of the chronic fibrosis process. At present, targeting chronic inflammation and oxidation seems to be a reasonable option to slow down renal fibrosis progression. Indeed, a number of experimental studies have demonstrated the efficiency of targeting inflammation and oxidative stress [14–17]. However, translation to the clinic is either missing or has been, most of the time, disappointing due to non-desirable side effects [14–17]. In addition, due to the chronicity of renal diseases one might wonder if a long-term specific anti-inflammatory treatment would promote susceptibility to infection. Taken together, it seems that targeting a single factor or pathway is not sufficient to efficiently prevent renal tubulointerstitial fibrosis. Therefore, it is understandable that a growing number of studies have investigated the health benefit of traditional medicine, also called natural/herbal medicine, including medicinal plants, which can be considered as a "multidrug" therapy. However, regarding the use of herbal medicine in the prevention and treatment of CKD, and more precisely tubulointerstitial fibrosis, very few studies have been carried out mainly due to the dramatic consequences associated with the ingestion of Chinese herbal medicine containing aristolochic acid [18,19]. It is thus very important to perform rigorous preclinical investigations to assess the presence of nephrotoxic molecules, as well as the beneficial and/or deleterious/toxic effects of these plants/molecules, particularly in the context of kidney disease.

In Reunion Island, since 2012, 27 medicinal plants have been registered at the French pharmacopeia [20] (https://ansm.sante.fr/, accessed on 30 March 2021). Most of them are known for their antioxidant and anti-inflammatory activities related mostly to their polyphenols content. However, although a number of studies (mostly in vitro studies) have reported various potential therapeutic effects such as antihypertensive [21], antioxidant, anti-inflammatory [22], antiviral [23], antiplasmodial and anti-Chikungunya effects [24], as well as an inhibitory effect on Dengue and Zika virus infection [25], the in vivo validation phase for further medical uses of these effects on preclinical models is missing.

Antirhea borbonica (*A. borbonica*) leaves are peculiarly interesting, as they are widely used in traditional medicine for treating, among others, diabetes, urinary tract infection, diarrhea, hemorrhage, rheumatism and also kidney stones [26,27]. Our laboratory has shown that *A. borbonica* exhibited strong antioxidant and anti-inflammatory effects, in vitro, on preadipocytes, cerebral endothelial cells and red blood cells [22,28,29]. Those antioxidant and anti-inflammatory biological effects were mainly associated with the capacity of polyphenols to down-regulate on one hand key molecular targets such as IL6, MCP-1 and NF-kB, and on the other hand increase superoxide dismutase (SOD) as well as the redox-sensitive translational factor Nrf2. In addition, the in vitro studies showed that predominant polyphenols such as quercetin, chlorogenic and caffeic acids were able to reduce free radicals through DPPH and AAPH radical-scavenging tests [22,28,29].

More recent data obtained in vivo also highlight a preventive protective effect of *A. borbonica* aqueous extract in a zebrafish diet-induced overweight model in displaying cerebral oxidative stress and blood–brain barrier leakage [30], as well as in a mouse stroke model [31]. Registration at the French pharmacopeia supposes that the medicinal plants are devoid of toxic effects in humans. Most of the time, this statement is based on ethnobotany investigations, mainly oral information/folk knowledge, claiming that the consumption of the plant is free from toxicities and side effects. However, regarding *A. borbonica*, to the best of our knowledge, no in vivo preclinical study investigating a putative nephroprotective effect has been reported. We have recently reported a detailed (qualitative and quantitative) phenolic profile as well as the antioxidant activity of aqueous and organic extracts of *A. borbonica* and determined the LC_{50} of both extracts on a zebrafish embryos model [32] according to the OECD (Organisation for Economic Co-operation and Develpoment) guidelines, allowing us to safely investigate in vivo the effect of *A. borbonica* in a kidney disease context.

Because of the potential therapeutic interest of *A. borbonica* against renal tubulointerstitial fibrosis, but also because we have previously reported [32] that the main polyphenols of *A. borbonica* was caffeic acid (CA) and since it is now well admitted that the absorption of CA derivatives results in free CA as secondary metabolites [33], the aims of our study were (i) to look for the presence of nephrotoxic molecules, (ii) to evaluate the renal antifibrotic effect of *A. borbonica* as well as CA in the in vivo unilateral ureteral obstruction (UUO) mouse model and (iii) to investigate the presence of putative specific antifibrotic molecules from *A. borbonica* at the renal tissue level.

2. Materials and Methods

2.1. Chemicals and Reagents

Folin–Ciocalteu reagent, sodium carbonate, sodium nitrite, aluminum chloride, 2,2-Diphenyl-1-picrylhydrazyl (DPPH) and caffeic acid (CA) were purchased from Sigma Aldrich (St. Louis, MO, USA). Solvents such as acetone, acetonitrile and methanol were purchased from Carlo Erba (Peypin, France).

2.2. Plant Material

Antirhea borbonica J.F Gmelin (*A. borbonica*) powder prepared from the dried leaves was obtained from the APLAMEDOM institute (Association pour les Plantes Aromatiques et Médicinales de la Réunion) and registered under the following code: DéTROI.002/2018, stating the date of collection and the GPS coordinates (21°05′44.9″ S, 55°39′06.6″ E), altitude: 770 m. The pharmacist and director of APLAMEDOM performed the botanical identification of *A. borbonica*. *A. borbonica* powder was stored at −20 °C until polyphenol extraction.

2.3. Nephrotoxic Compounds Identification and Quantification of Polyphenols by UPLC-UV-ESI-MS/MS

Polyphenolic extract from *A. borbonica* was prepared by dissolving 1 g of crushed leaves in 25 mL of an aqueous acetonic solution (70%, v/v). After incubation at 4 °C for 90 min, the mixture was centrifuged at $3500 \times g$ rpm at 4 °C for 20 min and polyphenol-rich supernatant was collected and stored at −80 °C until analysis. Identification of polyphenols was carried out by ultra-high-performance liquid chromatography (UHPLC) coupled with diode array detection and a HESI-Orbitrap mass spectrometer (Q Exactive Plus, Thermo Fisher). A 10 µL sample volume was injected using an UHPLC system equipped with a Thermo Fisher Ultimate 3000 series WPS-3000 RS autosampler and then separated on a PFP column (2.6 µm, 100 mm × 2.1 mm, Phenomenex, Torrance, CA, USA). The column was eluted with a gradient mixture of 0.1% formic acid in water (A) and 0.1% formic acid in acetonitrile (B) at the flow rate of 0.450 mL/min, with 5% B at 0.00 to 0.1 min, 35% B at 0.1 to 7.1 min, 95% B at 7.2 to 7.9 min and 5% B at 8.0 to 10 min. The column temperature was held at 30 °C and the detection wavelengths were set to 280 and 310 nm.

For mass spectrometer conditions, a Heated Electrospray Ionization source II (HESI II) was used. Nitrogen was used as drying gas. The mass spectrometric conditions were optimized as follows: spray voltage = 2.8 kV, capillary temperature = 350 °C, sheath gas flow rate = 60 units, aux gas flow rate = 20 units and S lens RF level = 50. Mass spectra were registered in full scan mode from m/z 100 to 1500 in negative ion mode at a resolving power of 70,000 FWHM at m/z 400. The automatic gain control (AGC) was set at 1e6. The MS/MS spectra were obtained by applying a relatively higher energy collisional dissociation (HCD) energy of 25%.

Identification of the compounds of interest was based on their retention time, exact mass, elemental composition, MS fragmentation pattern and comparisons with available standards and the advanced mass spectral database, m/z Cloud (https://www.mzcloud.org, accessed on 3 February 2021). The search for nephrotoxic compounds was carried out based on their exact mass in the MS spectrum (Extract Ions Chromatograms (XICs)). Data were acquired by XCalibur 4.2 software (Thermo Fisher Scientific Inc., Waltham, MA, USA) and processed with compound discoverer 2.1, and Skyline 20.1 software (MacCoss Lab., Seattle, WA, USA) was used to confront raw files with our "in house" database.

2.4. Desorption Electrospray Ionization-High Resolution/Mass Spectrometry (DESI-HR/MS) Imaging

The 2D automated Omni Spray Kidney tissues were flash-frozen in nitrogen and stored at −80 °C before DESI-HR/MS imaging. For DESI-MS imaging and histology, 12 μm thickness kidney sections were collected and mounted on SuperFrost™ Plus glass slides.

The 2D automated Omni Spray ion source from Prosolia Inc. (Indianapolis, IN, USA) coupled to a Q-Exactive™ Plus mass spectrometer (Thermo Fisher Scientific, Bremen, Germany) was used to perform the mass spectrometry imaging experiment. A solution of methanol with 0.1% formic acid (HPLC-MS grade, Carlo Erba) was used as the extraction and ionization spray solvent, delivered by a syringe pump at a flow rate of 5 μL/min. All imaging experiments were carried out with the following experimental conditions including source parameters: 2.8 kV capillary voltage, 250 °C capillary temperature, 60% S-lens RF level and 86 psi nitrogen nebulizing gas pressure, and including geometrical parameters: ∼1 mm spray tip-to-surface distance and a spray incident angle of 60°. Mass spectra were registered in full scan mode with the mass spectrometer operating in negative mode. Survey full scan mass spectra were acquired in the 50 to 500 m/z range at resolving power 70,000 (at m/z 400) with an automatic gain control (AGC) target of 3^6 and maximum injection time of 200 ms. DESI-HR/MS imaging of tissues was performed in start point-constant velocity scan mode, with a scan rate of 185.2 μm/s and a spatial resolution of 100 μm. Mass spectra were acquired using XCalibur 4.2 software (Thermo Fisher Scientific Inc.).The XCalibur mass spectral files (.raw) were converted to mZML then to imzML [34]. MSIQuant software [35] was used to generate the selected ion images.

Periodic acid-Schiff (PAS) staining was performed on the same tissue sections after DESI-MSI to visualize tissue structure.

2.5. Animal Model: Unilateral Ureteral Obstruction (UUO)—Biodistribution and Pharmacokinetic Studies

All reported experiments were performed at the GIP-CYROI technological platform's animal facility (A974001), conducted in accordance with NIH guidelines for the care and use of laboratory animals, and were approved by the French authorities (APAFIS#7347-2016100314466830v5, approved on 4 September 2017). C57BL/6J mice (male, 6 weeks old) were purchased from Janvier, (Le Genest Saint Isle, France) and housed in a pathogen-free, temperature-controlled environment with a 12–12 h light/dark photocycle. Animals had free access to food and tap water, to avoid dehydration-related hypovolemia. All mice were fed with a normal diet.

The unilateral ureteral ligation was performed as previously described [36]. Briefly, under oxygen–isoflurane anesthesia and through a longitudinal, left abdominal incision, the ureter was exposed and ligated with a 6/0 nylon thread at the uretero–pelvic junction. In sham operations, the ureter was exposed but not ligated and repositioned. To reduce pain Buprenorphine (0.01 mg/kg) (Buprecare centravet, Maison-Alfort, France) was injected i.p before surgery and 12 h later. Except for the preventive experiment where *A. borbonica* polyphenol-rich extract was administered by gavage 1 day before UUO and then every day for 5 days, the treatment with *A. borbonica* polyphenol extract (25 mg/kg) or CA (25 mg/kg) was initiated 3 days after UUO and continued for 5 days. *A. borbonica* polyphenol extract (25 mg/kg) or CA (25 mg/kg) were resuspended in distilled water just before gavage. The control group received only the vehicle (distilled water). At the end of the different protocols, mice were sacrificed and the kidneys were removed, and a transverse section was fixed in Carnoy's solution for 24 h and subsequently embedded in paraffin for immunohistological analysis. Several pieces of renal cortex were snap-frozen in liquid nitrogen and stored at −80 °C for mRNA, enzyme activities and MS/MS analysis.

For biodistribution study, one day before sacrifice animals were placed in metabolic cages to collect urine overnight. CA and its metabolites were measured by UPLC-MS/MS in liver and kidney tissues and urine.

For pharmacokinetics study, the animals were submitted to UUO and 3 days later they were fasted overnight and then treated with a single dose of CA (25 mg/kg) or vehicle (n = 3/group). Blood samples (90 µL) were collected at time 0 (before treatment), 30 min, 60 min, 180 min and 360 min post-treatment. CA concentrations were measured by UPLC-HESI-Q-orbitrap (Q Exactive Plus).

2.6. Determination of Phenolic and Flavonoid Contents—Measurement of the Total Antioxidant Capacity of Polyphenol-Rich Plant Extract Administered Orally

The total phenolic acid content in *A. borbonica* extract was determined by using the Folin–Ciocalteu assay [37] and expressed as mg gallic acid equivalent (GAE) per 100 g dry plant powder. The total flavonoid content was determined by using the aluminum chloride ($AlCl_3$) colorimetric assay [38] and expressed as mg quercetin equivalent (QE) per 100 g dry plant powder.

The total antioxidant capacity of *A. borbonica* extract was assessed through the 2,2-Diphenyl-1-picrylhydrazyl (DPPH) radical scavenging assay using vitamin C positive control. The absorbance (Abs) was read at 517 nm (FLUOstar Optima, Bmg Labtech). The percentage of free radical-quenching activity of DPPH was calculated from the following formula:

$$\text{Antioxidant capacity (\%)} = [(Abs_{vehicle} - Abs_{sample})/Abs_{vehicle}] \times 100$$

2.7. Immunohistochemistry and Histological Analysis

Kidneys were fixed in Carnoy's solution, dehydrated and embedded in paraffin. From kidney sections, routine histology and immunohistological staining and analysis were performed as previously described [39]. Three to four µm thickness sections were cut and used for routine staining (hematoxylin–eosin and Sirius red staining) and immunohistochemistry. The extent of Sirius red staining on the kidney section was scored from 0 to 4+ as follows: 0: no staining; 0.5: <10%; 1: 10–25%; 2: 25–50%; 3: 50–75%; and 4: >75%. For immunohistochemistry, mouse renal tissue was first de-waxed in toluene and rehydrated through a series of graded ethanol washes before incubation with 3% hydrogen peroxide for 10 min at room temperature to block endogenous peroxidase activity. Specific primary antibodies were incubated (1 h at room temperature) on mouse kidney sections for the detection of macrophages with anti-mouse F4/80 (RM2900; Caltag laboratories Inc., Burlingame, CA, USA; dilution 1/250); rabbit anti-alpha smooth muscle actin antibodies (ab5694-abcam; dilution 1/250). The sections were subsequently stained with the Dako Envision system (K4000 (primary antibodies from mouse) and K4002 (primary antibodies from rabbit)) according to manufacturer's instruction. Sections were finally counterstained with hematoxylin. Negative controls for the immunohistochemical procedures included substitution of the primary antibody with nonimmune sera at a similar immunoglobin concentration. Sections were scanned using a NanoZoomer S60 (Hamamatsu) and image analysis was realized in a blind fashion using Image J software (https://imagej.nih.gov/ij/, accessed on 30 March 2021).

2.8. RT-qPCR

Total RNA was isolated from mouse kidneys with TRIzol™ reagent (Invitrogen). One microgram of total RNA was reverse transcribed with random hexamer primers and Superscript II reverse transcriptase (Applied Biosystems). The quantitative real-time polymerase chain reaction was performed in a 96 well plate using SYBR green™ master mix (Eurogentec). Analysis of GAPDH was performed to normalize gene expression and the relative mRNA fold changes between groups were calculated using the $2^{-\Delta\Delta Ct}$ method. Primer sequences are listed in Table 1.

Table 1. Primers used for reverse transcribed-quantitative polymerase chain reaction (RT-qPCR). Transforming growth Figure 4. nuclear factor erythroid 2-related factor 2 (*Nrf2*); monocyte chemotactic protein (*Mcp1*); fibronectin (*Fn*); collagen type I and III (*Col I, Col III*); alpha smooth muscle actin (*α-Sma*); catalase (*Cat*); glutathione peroxidase (*Gpx*); manganese-dependent superoxide dismutase (*MnSOD*); copper/zinc superoxide dismutase (*Cu/ZnSOD*).

Mouse Gene	Sequence	
Tgf-β	Forward	CCTGAGTGGCTGTCTTTTGA
	Reverse	CGTGGAGTTTGTTATCTTTGCTG
Tnf-α	Forward	TCCCAGGTTCTCTTCAAGGGA
	Reverse	ACAAGGTACAACCCATCGGC
Nf-κB	Forward	GTGATGGGCCTTCACACACA
	Reverse	CATTTGAACACTGCTTTGACT
F4/80	Forward	ACCACAATACCTACATGCACC
	Reverse	AAGCAGGCGAGGAAAAGATAG
Nrf2	Forward	TCCCATTTGTAGATGACCATGAG
	Reverse	CCATGTCCTGCTCTATGCTG
Mcp1	Forward	GCAGTTAACGCCCCACTCA
	Reverse	CCAGCCTACTCATTGGGATCA
Fn	Forward	CTTTGGCAGTGGTCATTTCAG
	Reverse	ATTCTCCCTTTCCATTCCCG
Col I	Forward	CATAAAGGGTCATCGTGGCT
	Reverse	TTGAGTCCGTCTTTGCCAG
Col III	Forward	GAAGTCTCTGAAGCTGATGGG
	Reverse	TTGCCTTGCGTGTTTGATATTC
α-Sma	Forward	GTGAAGAGGAAGACAGCACAG
	Reverse	GCCCATTCCAACCATTACTCC
Gapdh	Forward	CTTTGTCAAGCTCATTTCCTGG
	Reverse	TCTTGCTCAGTGTCCTTGC
Cat	Forward	CCTCCTCGTTCAGGATGTGGTT
	Reverse	CGAGGGTCACGAACTGTGTCAG
Gpx	Forward	TGCTCATTGAGAATGTCGCGTCTC
	Reverse	AGGCATTCCGCAGGAAGGTAAAGA
MnSod	Forward	ATGTTGTGTCGGGCGGCG
	Reverse	AGGTAGTAAGCGTGCTCCCACACG
Cu/ZnSod	Forward	GCAGGGAACCATCCACTT
	Reverse	TACAACCTCTGGACCCGT

2.9. Protein Isolation from Kidney Tissue, Antioxidant Activities (Mn-SOD, Cu/Zn-SOD, GPX, CAT) and Protein Carbonylation

For enzymatic activities determination, protein isolation from kidney tissue was performed as follow: between 10 to 30 mg of kidney tissues previously collected and stored at −80 °C were homogenized with a TissueLyser II (Qiagen) in 150 μL of Tris buffer (Tris (25 mM), EDTA (1 mM), pH 7.4). After centrifugation (5000× *g*/min, for 10 min), the supernatant was used for protein quantification and enzymatic assays. The total protein level of lysate was quantified by the bicinchoninic acid assay (BCA).

SOD activity was assayed by monitoring the rate of acetylated cytochrome c reduction by superoxide radicals generated by the xanthine/xanthine oxidase system. Measurements were performed in a reagent buffer (xanthine oxidase, xanthine (0.5 mM), cytochrome c (0.2 mM), KH_2PO_4 (50 mM), EDTA (2 mM), pH 7.8) at 25 °C. The specific MnSOD activities were determined in the same conditions after incubation of samples with NaCN (1 mM) which inhibits Cu/ZnSOD activities. Assays were monitored by spectrophotometry at 560 nm. SOD activities were calculated using a calibration standard curve of SOD (up to 6 unit/mg). Total SOD, MnSOD and resulting Cu/ZnSOD activities were expressed as international catalytic units per mg of proteins.

The total activity of glutathione peroxidase (GPX) was determined with cumene hydroperoxide as substrate. The rate of glutathione oxidized by cumene hydroperoxide (6.5 mM) was evaluated by the decrease in NADPH (0.12 mM in Tris buffer) at 340 nm in the presence of NaCN (10 mM), reduced glutathione (0.25 mM) and glutathione reductase (1 U/mL) in Tris buffer (50 mM, pH 8). GPX activity was expressed as international units per gram of proteins.

The catalase (CAT) activity assay was carried out on 40 µg of protein lysate in 25 mM Tris–HCl (pH 7.5). Blanks were measured at 240 nm just before adding 80 µL of H_2O_2 (10 mM final) to start the reaction. Catalase activity was determined by measuring the absorbance at 240 nm and was calculated using a calibration standard curve of an increasing amount of catalase between 12.5 and 125 unit/mL. Catalase activity was expressed as international catalytic units per mg of proteins.

The protein carbonylation was determined as described previously [40] by the carbonyl ELISA assay based on the recognition of protein-bound DNPH in carbonylated proteins with an anti-DNP antibody.

2.10. Statistics

Individual data are presented as dot plots next to the average for the group. Comparison between two groups of values was achieved by using a two-tailed unpaired Welch's t-test. For statistical comparisons involving more than two experimental groups, analysis of variance (ANOVA) followed by Dunnett's test was used. Statistical analyses and the determination of the area under the curve ($AUC_{(0-360)}$) were performed with Graph-Pad Prism 6.3 (GraphPad Software, Inc., San Diego, CA, USA). Data are mean ± SD. A p-value < 0.05 was considered statistically significant.

3. Results

3.1. Detection and Identification of Nephrotoxic Components

In the present study, based on their exact mass in MS spectrum, we focused on the detection and identification of known nephrotoxic molecules (Table S1) in the polyphenol-rich plant extract from *A. borbonica*. None of these molecules were found in the *A. borbonica* extract. This reassuring result prompts us to investigate, in vivo, the putative nephroprotective effect of a non-toxic concentration of polyphenol-rich extract from *A. borbonica*.

3.2. Phenolic/Flavonoid Contents and Total Antioxidant Activity of Orally Administered Polyphenol-Rich Extract from A. borbonica.

Based on our previous study [32], the dose of 25 mg/kg was chosen for mice gavage and corresponded to the lowest dose (1.4 g/L) tested on the zebrafish (embryos/larvae) model, showing no toxicological effect. As shown in Figure 1A, the quantity of polyphenol administered by gavage is not negligible since we found total contents of phenolic acids and flavonoids of 47.6 ± 8.5 mg GAE/100 g dried powder and of 27.1 ± 3.2 mg QE/100 g dried powder, respectively. In addition, *A. borbonica* extract exhibited an antioxidant capacity accounting for 37% of the positive control ascorbic acid (Figure 1B).

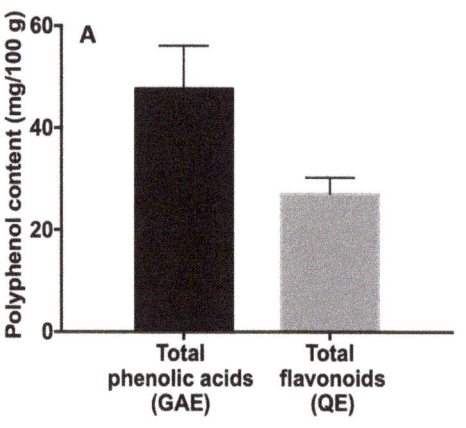 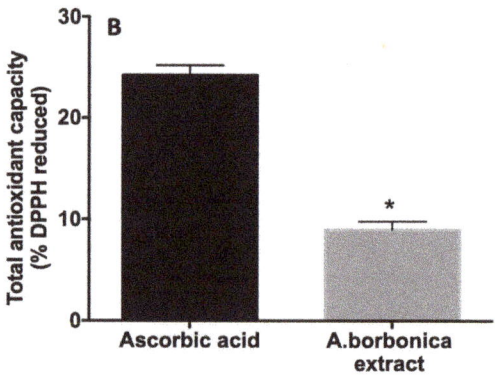

Figure 1. Total phenolic acid and flavonoid contents (**A**) and antioxidant capacity (**B**), from *A. borbonica* extract administered by gavage. (**A**) Total phenolic contents were determined by using the Folin–Ciocalteu colorimetric assay and total flavonoid contents were determined by using the aluminum chloride colorimetric assay. The results are expressed as mg gallic acid equivalent (GAE)/100 g and as mg quercetin equivalent (QE)/100 g plant dried powder. (**B**) Total antioxidant capacity was measured by DPPH assay. Positive control ascorbic acid was used at the same phenolic acid concentration (47 mg GAE) as that provided by the *A. borbonica* extract. The results are expressed as % of reduced DPPH. Data are means ± SD of three independent experiments. * $p < 0.05$ vs. ascorbic acid.

3.3. Preventive Experiment: Effects of Polyphenol-Rich Extract from A. borbonica on Body and Kidney Weight and Diuresis in a UUO Model

In order to ascertain that the 5 days of treatment with *A. borbonica* (25 mg/kg) did not result in unexpected adverse effects, we investigated the body weight before and after the treatments, and the diuresis and the left kidney weight at the end of the experiments. As shown in Table 2, neither the UUO treatment nor the UUO + *A. borbonica* treatment led to a significant change in animal body weight, kidney weight and diuresis.

Table 2. Effect of *A. borbonica* (*A. b*) extract on body weight, left kidney weight and diuresis. Values are means ± SD; $n = 7$ animals/group.

Group	n	Body Weight (g)	Left Kidney Weight (g)	Diuresis/24 h (mL)
Sham	7	22.02 ± 2.64	0.134 ± 0.01	1.06 ± 0.44
UUO + veh	7	21.58 ± 1.54	0.136 ± 0.01	1.26 ± 0.6
UUO + *A. b* 25 mg/kg	7	20.49 ± 1.20	0.122 ± 0.008	1.06 ± 0.6

3.4. Preventive Effect of Polyphenol-Rich Extract from A. borbonica in UUO-Induced Tubulointerstitial Fibrosis

To determine the possible nephroprotective effect of polyphenol-rich extract from *A. borbonica*, we administrated it by gavage one day before the UUO and allowed the mice to survive for 5 days with a daily *A. borbonica* gavage. The sham group received the vehicle (distilled water). At the end of the experimental procedure (day 5), we assessed interstitial collagen deposition by the analysis of Sirius red-stained renal sections (Figure 2A). In this "proof of concept" study, identification of a nephroprotective effect leads us to pursue the investigation, otherwise we do not go any further.

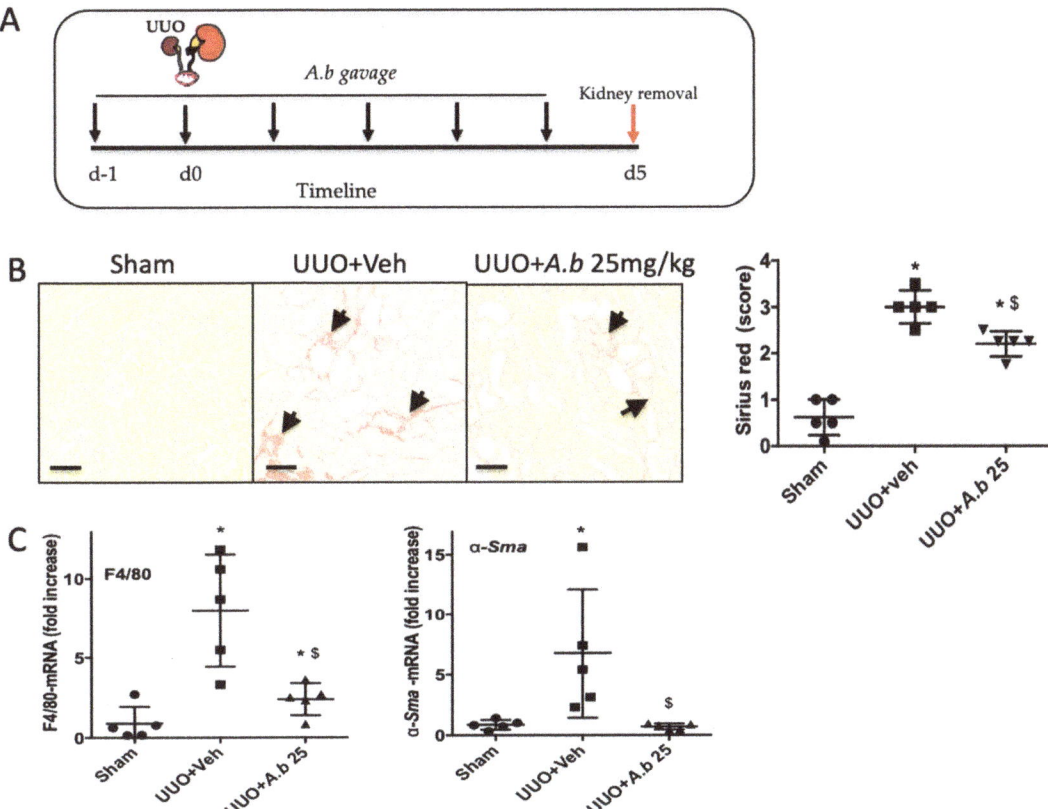

Figure 2. Preventive effect of *A. borbonica* (*A. b*) 25 mg/kg on renal tubulointerstitial fibrosis induced by unilateral ureteral obstruction (UUO) in mice. (**A**) Experiment design: black arrows indicate daily gavage with 25 mg/kg *A. b*. (**B**) Renal tubulointerstitial fibrosis highlighted with the Sirius red staining, arrows indicate interstitial fibrosis. (**C**) qPCR analyses of mRNA–macrophage infiltration (F4/80) and myofibroblasts (α-Sma); n = 5 per group. * $p < 0.05$ compared to Sham; \$ $p < 0.05$ compared to UUO + Veh. Scale bar =100 µm.

Pretreatment with polyphenol-rich extract from *A. borbonica* (25 mg/kg) for 5 days significantly decreased tubulointerstitial collagen accumulation as shown by the Sirius red staining (Figure 2B). Because interstitial collagen accumulation is strongly associated with an increase in macrophage infiltration (F4/80) in the kidney and the appearance of myofibroblasts (α-SMA), we examined the mRNA expression of these two markers. Whereas UUO increased the gene expression of *F4/80* and *α-SMA*, both markers were significantly decreased in the group treated with polyphenol-rich extract from *A. borbonica* (Figure 2C).

This very first experiment performed on a reduced number of animals and the rapid evaluation of the three phases of the fibrotic process (inflammation, myofibroblasts appearance and interstitial collagens accumulation) allowed us to make the decision to continue the evaluation of the polyphenol-rich extract from *A. borbonica*.

3.5. Curative Effect of Polyphenol-Rich Extract from A. borbonica in UUO-Induced Tubulointerstitial Fibrosis.

To truly evaluate the nephroprotective effect of polyphenol-rich extract from *A. borbonica*, we administered the solution, by gavage, 3 days after surgery for 5 days (Figure 3A). *A. borbonica* extract significantly reduced macrophage infiltration and myofibroblast appearance, assessed by F4/80 (Figure 3B) and α−SMA (Figure 3C) immunostaining, respectively, and confirmed by qPCR analysis. Moreover, *A. borbonica* extract decreased extracellular matrix accumulation assessed by Sirius red staining (Figure 3D).

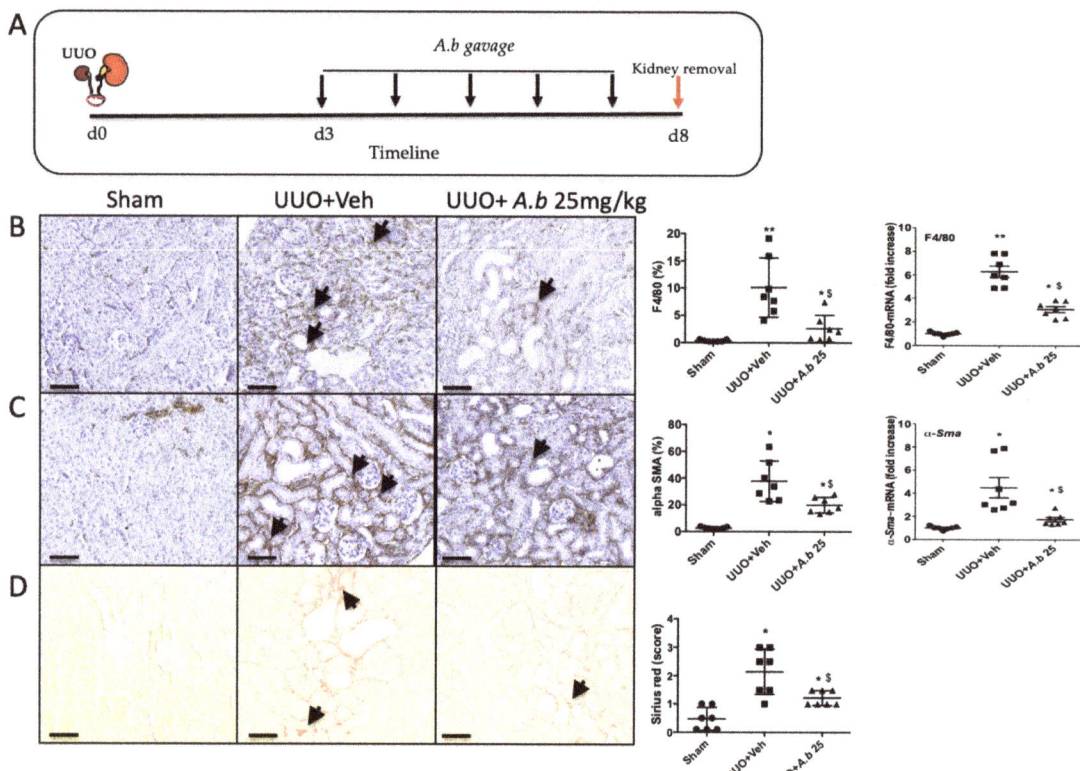

Figure 3. Curative effect of *A. borbonica* (*A. b*) 25 mg/kg on renal tubulointerstitial fibrosis induced by unilateral ureteral obstruction (UUO) in mice. (**A**) Experiment design: the black arrows indicate daily gavage with *A. b*. (**B**) Macrophage infiltration revealed by F4/80 immunostaining, arrows indicate macrophages. (**C**) Accumulation of myofibroblasts revealed by alpha SMA staining, arrows indicate myofibroblasts. (**D**) Renal tubulointerstitial fibrosis shown by Sirius red staining, arrows indicate interstitial fibrosis. Sham-operated group (Sham), unilateral ureteral obstruction group receiving vehicle (UUO + Veh) and unilateral ureteral obstruction group receiving polyphenol-rich extract from *A. b* (UUO + *A. b* 25 mg/kg). For each staining, quantitative results are shown on the right part of the figure (scatter dot plot), as well as renal mRNA expression of *F4/80* and *α-Sma*; n = 7 per group. * $p < 0.05$, ** $p < 0.01$, compared to Sham; $ $p < 0.05$ compared to UUO + Veh. Scale bar = 100 µm.

To better understand the molecular mechanisms by which *A. borbonica* could reduce renal fibrosis, we analyzed the expression of genes encoding key proteins known to be involved in UUO. Shown in Figure 4A is the UUO-induced overexpression of the mRNA of profibrotic cytokines (*TGF-β*, *TNF-α*) and *NF-κB*, a nuclear factor known to control cytokines production. We also observed the overexpression of *Nrf2*, a redox-sensitive nuclear transcription factor involved in the regulation of antioxidant enzyme genes expression. The mRNA *Mcp-1* encoding for the chemokine MCP-1 (also known as CCL2) which is involved in monocyte/macrophage recruitment was overexpressed by UUO. As expected, UUO induced the expression of fibronectin, type I and III interstitial collagens' mRNA. Oral administration of *A. borbonica* extract blunted significantly the UUO-induced expression of most of these genes. Interestingly, *A. borbonica* extract induced a significant increase in the mRNA expression of *Nrf2*, suggesting the stimulation of the antioxidant defense system.

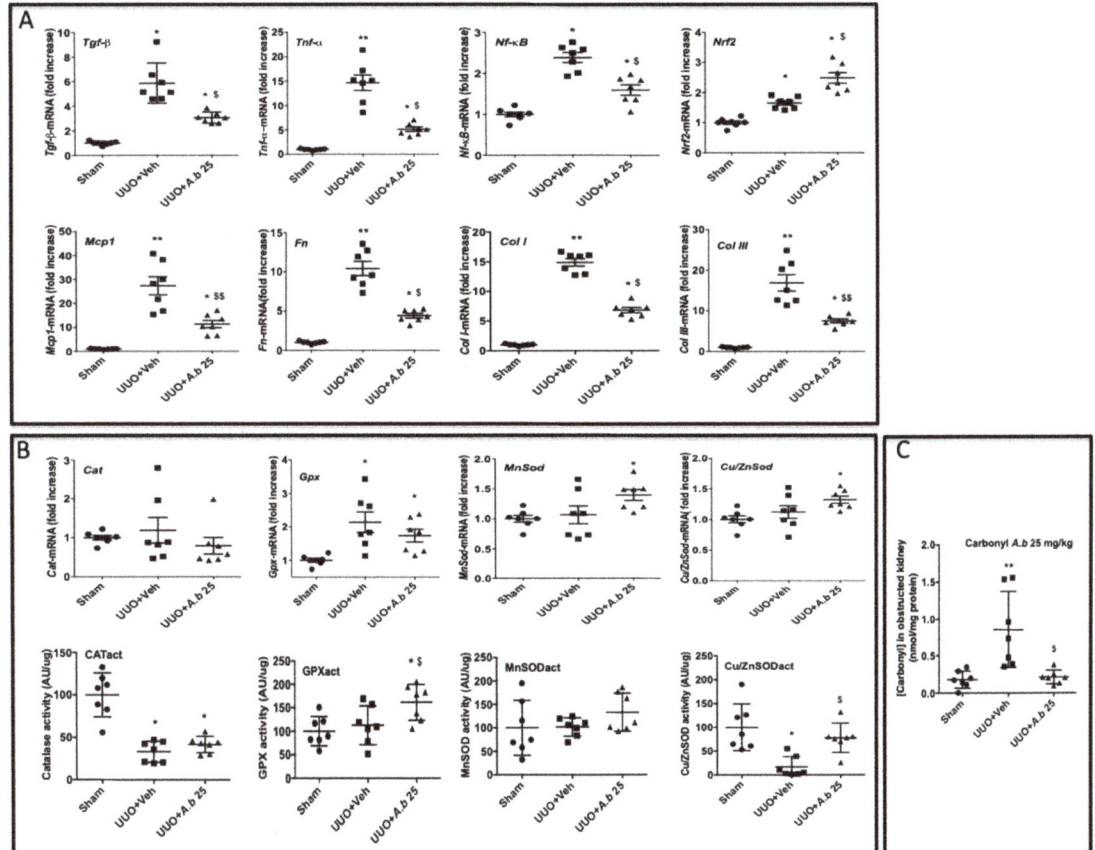

Figure 4. *A. borbonica* (*A. b*) extract restores normal inflammatory and oxidative stress states induced by unilateral ureteral obstruction (UUO). (**A**) Expression of genes involved in inflammatory and fibrotic responses in obstructed kidney, (**B**) antioxidant enzyme expression and activity (act) and (**C**) protein carbonyl concentration in obstructed kidney. $n = 7$ per group. * $p < 0.05$, ** $p < 0.01$, compared to Sham; $^\$$ $p < 0.05$, $^{\$\$}$ $p < 0.01$ compared to UUO + Veh.

These results prompt us to investigate the gene expression and enzyme activities of catalase (CAT), glutathione peroxidase (GPX) and Mn- and Cu/Zn-superoxide dismutase (SOD). As shown in Figure 4B, gene expression did not change for *Cat*. *Gpx* was increased by UUO whereas *Mn-* and *Cu/Zn-SOD* expression was not modified when compared to the sham group. *A. borbonica* extract treatment significantly increased *Mn-* and *Cu/Zn-SOD* mRNA expression compared to the sham group, but this increase was not significant when compared to the UUO untreated group. Interestingly, we found that, when compared to the UUO group, *A. borbonica* extract treatment was associated with a significant increase in both GPX and Cu/Zn-SOD enzyme activities. More precisely, UUO did not change the GPX enzyme activity but significantly decreased Cu/Zn-SOD activity, and *A. borbonica* extract administration significantly increased GPX and brought back to control values Cu/Zn-SOD activities.

Protein carbonylation is considered as a major hallmark of oxidative damage. The disturbance of redox homeostasis in the UUO model could explain the significant increase in protein carbonyl level in obstructed kidneys, as shown in Figure 4C. Interestingly, this increase was totally suppressed by *A. borbonica* extract treatment (Figure 4C).

3.6. Biodistribution of Caffeic Acid and Its Metabolite 24 Hours after Administration of A. borbonica Polyphenol-Rich Extract (25 mg/kg) in Mice Kidney, Liver and Urine

In the next step, we aimed at evaluating the biodistribution of the main polyphenols of *A. borbonica* and caffeic acid derivatives by using mass spectrometry, in order to identify metabolites that may explain the previously observed biological effects. As shown in Table 3, the caffeic acid (CA) was detected as a secondary metabolite in the UUO animals treated with *A. borbonica* polyphenol extract, and was significantly higher in obstructed kidneys when compared to sham and vehicle groups (0.144 ± 0.013 vs. 0.006 ± 0.006 µM, respectively, *** $p < 0.001$). Similarly, significantly elevated concentrations of the methylated form of CA, namely ferulic acid (FA), were detected in the *A. borbonica*-treated UUO mice group (1.119 ± 0.132 vs. 0.076 ± 0.060/0.064 ± 0.011 µM, respectively, *** $p < 0.001$). No metabolite difference was noticed between each group for liver samples. Nonetheless, the highest concentrations of CA and FA were found in urine (96.599 ± 19.704 vs. 38.002 ± 5.021 µM, respectively), indicating excretion, at least in part, by the kidneys. As expected, *A. borbonica* polyphenols were detected in the liver. Caffeic acid and its secondary metabolite FA reach the systemic circulation to be delivered to organs. These findings prompt us to investigate the effect of the CA molecule in this kidney fibrosis model.

Table 3. Distribution of caffeic acid (CA) and its methylated metabolite, ferulic acid (FA), in obstructed kidney, liver and urine after ingestion of 25 mg/kg of *A. borbonica* (A. b). The concentrations were measured by UPLC-HESI-Q-Orbitrap (Q-Exactive™ Plus) and expressed in (µM). ** $p < 0.01$, *** $p < 0.001$, compared to UUO + Vehicle. Values are means ± SD; $n = 7$ animals/group.

Concentration (mM)	Sham	UUO + Vehicle	UUO + A. b 25 mg/kg
Kidney obstructed			
Caffeic acid	0.006 ± 0.005	0.006 ± 0.006	0.144 ± 0.013 ***
Ferulic acid	0.076 ± 0.060	0.064 ± 0.011	1.119 ± 0132 ***
Liver			
Caffeic acid	0.026 ± 0.006	0.031 ± 0.003	0.037 ± 0.001
Ferulic acid	0.391 ± 0.074	0.388 ± 0.104	0.426 ± 0.099
Urine			
Caffeic acid	24.912 ± 6.401	21.161 ± 6.856	96.599 ± 19.704 ***
Ferulic acid	10.376 ± 3.505	12.551 ± 3.307	38.002 ± 5.021 **

3.7. Caffeic Acid (CA) Administration Mimics A. borbonica Extract's Nephroprotective Effects

The presence of CA in mice obstructed kidney (Table 3) and the fact that CA and derivatives were the most abundant polyphenolic compounds of *A. borbonica* [32] suggests that CA could mimic *A. borbonica* extract's nephroprotective effects.

We thus investigated if we could reproduce the observed nephroprotective effects of *A. borbonica* by daily oral administration of CA from day 3 after UUO for 5 days (Figure 5A).

Immunohistological analysis showed a significant protective effect of CA on macrophage infiltration (Figure 5B), accumulation of myofibroblasts (Figure 5C) and renal tubulointerstitial fibrosis (Figure 5D). The overexpression of the mRNA levels of genes involved in the inflammatory and fibrotic responses in obstructed kidneys was downregulated by CA, except for the transcription factor *Nrf2* (Figure 6A), as previously described above for *A. borbonica*. We also observed that CA significantly increased CAT and Cu/ZnSOD enzyme activities (Figure 6B). However, the stimulation of the activity of these antioxidant enzymes by CA resulted in a slight decrease in carbonyl level which did not reach statistical significance (Figure 6C).

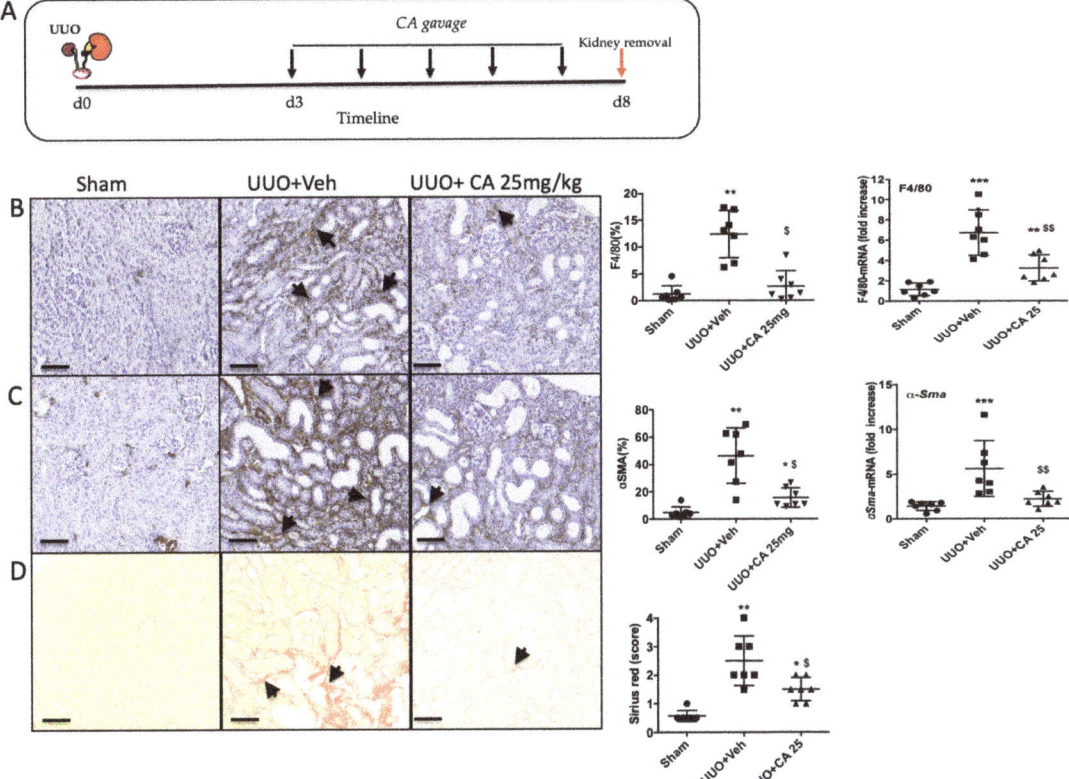

Figure 5. Curative effect of caffeic acid (CA) 25 mg/kg on renal tubulointerstitial fibrosis induced by UUO in mice. (**A**) Experiment design, black arrows indicate daily gavage with CA. (**B**) Macrophage infiltration F4/80, arrows indicate macrophages. (**C**) Accumulation of myofibroblasts alpha SMA, arrows indicate myofibroblasts. (**D**) Tubulointerstitial fibrosis (Sirius red), arrows indicate interstitial fibrosis. Sham operated group (Sham), unilateral ureteral obstruction group receiving vehicle (UUO + Veh) and unilateral ureteral obstruction group receiving caffeic acid (UUO + CA 25 mg/kg). For each staining quantitative results are shown on the right part of the figure (scatter dot plot), as well as renal mRNA expression of F4/80 and α-Sma; $n = 7$ per group. * $p < 0.05$, ** $p < 0.01$, *** $p < 0.001$, compared to Sham; $^\$ p < 0.05$, $^{\$\$} p < 0.01$ compared to UUO + Veh. Scale bar = 100 µm.

Taken together these data strongly suggest that the phenolic compound CA found in *A. borbonica.* could actively participate in the observed nephroprotective effects in the UUO model.

3.8. Plasma and Kidney Pharmacokinetic of Caffeic Acid

To evidence that CA participates in the nephroprotective effects of *A. borbonica* extract, we decided to undertake plasma and kidney pharmacokinetics of CA in order to optimize the visualization protocol of the CA presence in the obstructed kidneys by using DESI-HR/MS imaging. To this end, three days after UUO, mice were administrated by oral route a unique dose of CA (25 mg/kg) and then were sacrificed at 30, 60, 180 and 360 min. Caffeic acid (CA) and ferulic acid (FA) concentrations in both the plasma and kidney were assessed by using UPLC-HESI-Q-orbitrap (Q-Exactive™ Plus).

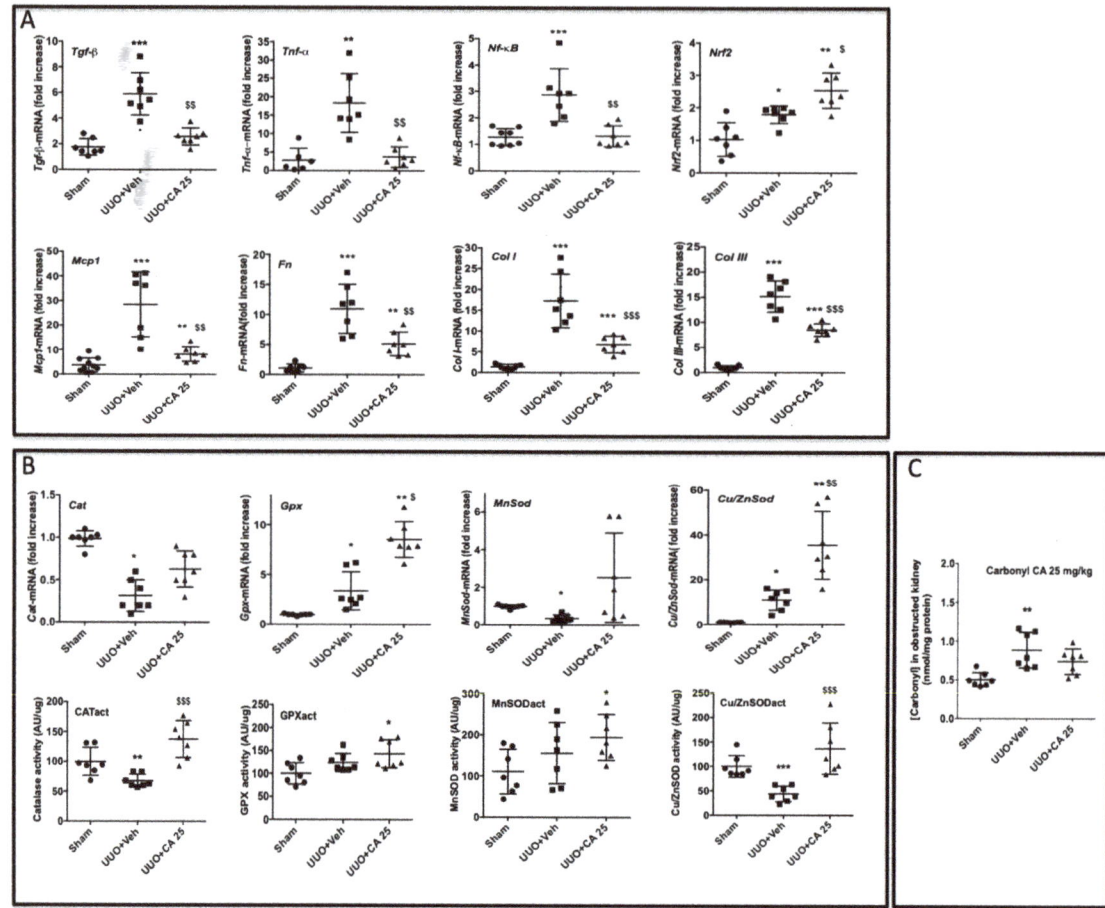

Figure 6. Caffeic acid (CA) 25 mg/kg restores normal inflammatory and oxidative stress parameters induced by UUO in mice. (**A**) Expression of genes involved in inflammatory and fibrotic responses in obstructed kidney, (**B**) antioxidant enzymes gene expression and activities and (**C**) the protein carbonyl concentration in obstructed kidney. $n = 7$ per group. * $p < 0.05$, ** $p < 0.01$, *** $p < 0.001$, compared to Sham; $ $p < 0.05$, $$ $p < 0.01$, $$$ $p < 0.001$, compared to UUO + Veh.

As shown in Figure 7A and Table 4, CA exhibited a significant peak plasma concentration of 50.5 ± 9.8 µM (C_{max}) within 30 min (t_{max}) suggesting its rapid absorption. However, due to hepatic first-pass metabolism, a limited bioavailability was noticed (0.4%). Indeed, a significant ferulic acid (FA) peak plasma concentration (68.3 ± 8.3 µM) appeared at the same t_{max} as CA. Comparison of the area under the curve (AUC) for plasma showed a significantly higher AUC $_{(0-360)}$ for CA than FA for UUO-CA treated mice (4964 ± 97.3 vs. 4648 ± 91.1, respectively), suggesting that CA stays longer in plasma than FA (Figure 7B). Notably, no plasma CA and FA peak was registered for the vehicle group. In the kidneys (Figure 7C,D), one hour after CA administration, CA and FA concentrations were significantly higher (x5) in the obstructed kidneys compared to the contralateral kidneys (5.3 ± 1.1 and 4.5 ± 0.8 µM vs. 0.3 ± 0.1 and 0.4 ± 0.1 µM, respectively). Interestingly, a significantly high AUC $_{(0-360)}$ was calculated for CA and FA in the obstructed kidneys compared to the contralateral kidneys (881 ± 17.2 and 1073 ± 21 vs. 100 ± 2 and 98.5 ± 11, respectively) indicating their accumulation in the obstructed kidney (Figure 7D). Taking these data into account we set up a DESI-HR/MS experiment to visualize the spatial distribution of CA in the obstructed kidney 1 h after CA gavage.

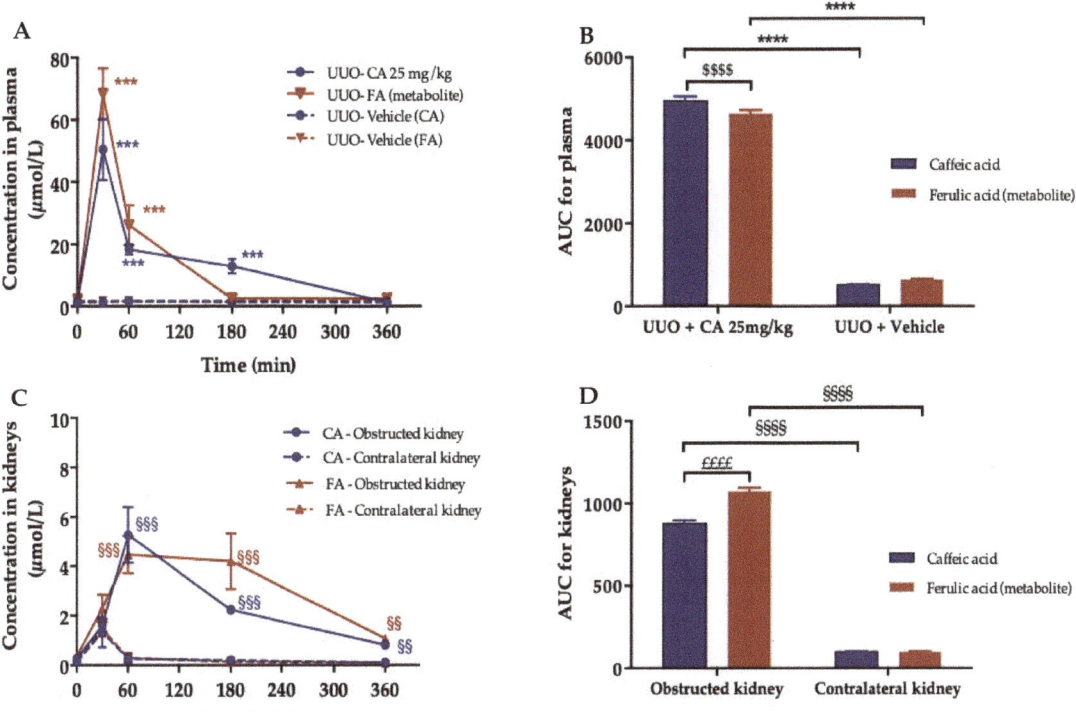

Figure 7. Pharmacokinetic study of caffeic acid (CA) and ferulic acid (FA) after oral administration of CA (25 mg/kg) in 3 days-UUO mice. (**A**) Plasma concentration–time profiles of CA and its circulation metabolite, ferulic acid (FA), in UUO mice. (**B**) Corresponding area under the curves (AUC) of CA and FA in plasma. (**C**) Concentration–time profiles of CA and FA in obstructed and contralateral kidneys. (**D**) Corresponding area under the curves (AUC) of CA and FA in obstructed and contralateral kidneys. Concentrations were determined using UPLC-HESI-Q-orbitrap (Q-Exactive™ Plus). *** $p < 0.001$, **** $p < 0.0001$, compared to UUO + Vehicle; $^{\$\$\$\$} p < 0.0001$, compared to caffeic acid; $^{\S\S} p < 0.01$, $^{\S\S\S} p < 0.001$, $^{\S\S\S\S} p < 0.0001$, compared to contralateral kidney; $^{££££} p < 0.0001$, compared to caffeic acid. Values are means ± SD; $n = 3$ animals/time.

Table 4. Pharmacokinetic parameters at the dose 25 mg/kg of caffeic acid (CA) orally administered in UUO mice. AUC represents the calculated area under the curve between 0 and 360 min. C_{max} is the maximum concentration achieved. t_{max} is the required time to achieve C_{max}. Bioavailability (F) is the fraction of the administered dose that is available to the systemic circulation. Values are means; $n = 3$ animals/time.

Parameter	Oral Administration (Gavage)
	Caffeic Acid
AUC $_{(0–360)}$	4964
C_{max} (µM)	50.5
t_{max} (min)	30
F (%)	0.4

3.9. Visualization of Orally Administered Caffeic Acid (CA) in the Obstructed Kidney

The spatial distribution of CA (m/z 179.0340) and FA (m/z 193.0506) in mice obstructed kidney is shown in Figure 8A,B respectively. When compared to PAS staining (Figure 8D) we observed the presence of CA in the renal cortex where the dilated tubules are found, and thus where tubulointerstitial fibrosis will appear and progress. Caffeic acid is also present in renal papilla, suggesting CA urinary elimination. Taken together our data highlight that CA exerts an antifibrotic effect in the UUO mouse model.

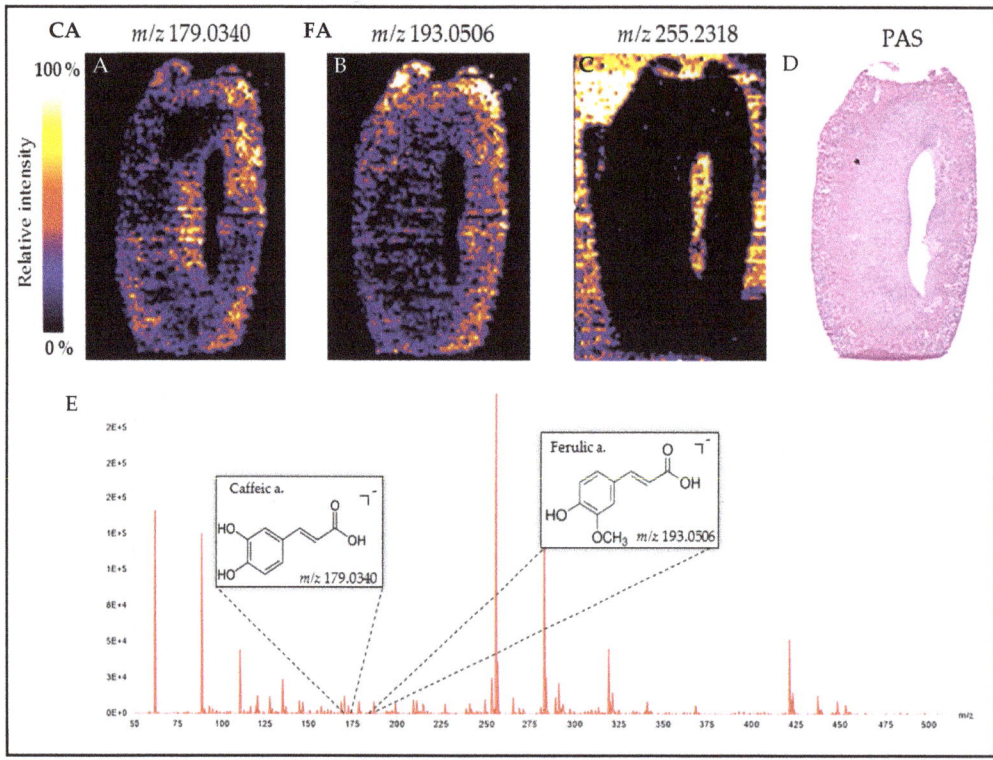

Figure 8. Visualization of caffeic acid (CA) and its circulating metabolite, ferulic acid (FA), 1 h post oral administration of CA 25 mg/kg in the obstructed kidney tissue of mice. Desorption electrospray ionization-high resolution/mass spectrometry (DESI-HR/MS) Imaging of (**A**) caffeic acid (m/z 179.0340), (**B**) ferulic acid (m/z 193.0506) and (**C**) m/z 255.2318 used to show the negative fingerprint of tissue and the corresponding Periodic Acid Schiff (PAS) staining (**D**). (**E**) DESI-HR/MS mass spectrum ranging from m/z 50 to 500. The Synapt Blue-Red-Yellow color scale was used.

4. Discussion

Medicinal plants are usually perceived as safe medication. However, plants can also contain many toxic substances that may be a risk to the kidneys [41,42]. Here, we first looked for the presence of known nephrotoxic molecules and showed that no toxic molecule, at least associated with Chinese herbal nephrotoxicity [43], was present in *A. borbonica*. These results made us confident to investigate in vivo the putative nephroprotective effect of *A. borbonica*.

Although rarely found in humans, the complete obstruction of the ureter in the UUO model mimics, in an accelerated manner, the different stages leading to renal tubulointerstitial fibrosis [44]. It includes inflammation associated with macrophage infiltration and the up-regulation of pro-fibrotic molecules, as well as the appearance and the accumulation of myofibroblasts, which are the main cell type responsible for the secretion of extracellular matrix proteins [44]. Because of the highly reproducible fibrotic response this UUO model is now well recognized to test the antifibrotic potency of candidate molecules [45].

In the present study, we provide evidence that the oral administration of polyphenol-rich extract from *A. borbonica* significantly attenuates, in vivo, renal interstitial fibrosis. We showed that this nephroprotective effect goes through reduction in the three phases of the fibrosis process (macrophage infiltration, myofibroblast appearance and extracellular matrix accumulation). An increasing number of studies using the UUO model have reported similar effects, mainly observed in a preventive way, from polyphenol-rich extracts of various origins such as *Elsholtzia ciliate* [46] and *Nigella sativa* [47], but also from polyphenol molecules such as curcumin from *Curcuma longa* [48], icariin, an active flavonoid from the *Epinedium* genus [49], resveratrol [50], quercetin, a flavonoid present in vegetables and fruits [51], and epigallocatechin-3-gallate, a green tea polyphenol [52]. In line with these studies, our results show, for the first time, that either in a preventive or curative treatment *A. borbonica* significantly attenuates macrophage infiltration. This anti-inflammatory effect leads to a strong decrease in myofibroblast appearance in the tubulointerstitial space and consequently to a reduced tubulointerstitial fibrosis, as evidenced by the down-regulation of *Fn* mRNA, as well as *Col I* and *III* at the mRNA and protein levels. As expected, this was associated with the mRNA down-regulation of pro-inflammatory and pro-fibrotic cytokines (*Tgf-β*, *Tnf-α*), a chemokine (*Mcp1*), and a transcription factor (*Nf-κB*).

As polyphenols are known to exert antioxidant effects [53], we studied the expression of *Nrf2*, which is a major transcription factor involved in the regulation of antioxidant enzymes [54,55]. We found that UUO induced an increase in *Nrf2* gene expression. This up-regulation was expected since UUO is known to induce oxidative stress [56], which in turn stimulates Nrf2 gene and protein expression [57]. In addition, we observed that polyphenol-rich extract from *A. borbonica* further stimulated *Nrf2* gene expression. It suggests that polyphenols from *A. borbonica* have the capacity to stimulate *Nrf2*. This result was consistent with the, now well admitted, effect of polyphenols such as Nrf2 activator [58]. To further get insights into the nephroprotective mechanism of polyphenol-rich extract from *A. borbonica*, we measured antioxidant enzymes known to be up-regulated by Nrf2. Whereas polyphenol-rich extract from *A. borbonica* was without significant effect on the mRNA expression of *Cat*, *Gpx* and *Sod* when compared to the UUO-untreated animals, we observed a significant increase in the enzyme activities of GPX and Cu/ZnSOD. Although most of the studies using the UUO model to investigate the renal effects of polyphenols have focused on the protein expression of antioxidant enzymes [49,59], our data are consistent with the few works that investigated the antioxidant enzyme activity, showing that the renal enzyme activities of CAT and total-SOD are significantly reduced in the obstructed kidney [47,60]. The decrease in these main antioxidant activities in the UUO model are generally associated with an increase in reactive oxygen species which can lead to protein damage and the formation of oxidized compounds such as carbonylated proteins [61]. Whereas polyphenol-rich extract from *A. borbonica* had no effect on CAT and Mn-SOD enzyme activities, our data show a significant increase in GPX and Cu/ZnSOD enzyme activities. These results specify more clearly the mechanism of action of *A. borbonica*. In addition, the beneficial effect of *A. borbonica* on both enzymes' activities seems to be strong enough to protect proteins from the oxidative damage induced by UUO.

We have previously reported [32] that CA and derivatives were the most abundant polyphenolic compounds of *A. borbonica*. In order to explore the mechanism of action of polyphenol-rich extract from *A. borbonica*, we investigated if we could reproduce the observed curative nephroprotective effects of *A. borbonica* extract by oral administration of CA. It is now well known that CA exhibits antioxidant and anti-inflammatory properties [62], and that administration of caffeamide derivatives have shown antifibrotic effects in renal ischemia reperfusion [63], as well as in the UUO model [64]. However, to the best of our knowledge, the oral administration of the CA molecule has never been studied in the UUO model. Since CA is the main phenolic acid found in *A. borbonica* [32], to properly investigate if CA participates in the antioxidant and anti-fibrotic effects observed with the polyphenol-rich extract from *A. borbonica*, we had to study the effect of oral administration of CA in the representative UUO renal tubulointerstitial fibrosis model. Our results clearly show that oral administration for 5 days of CA (25 mg/kg), 3 days after UUO, significantly decreased macrophage infiltration, myofibroblast appearance and extracellular matrix accumulation. This was associated with the down-regulation of pro-inflammatory and pro-fibrotic cytokines, as well as a significant increase in *Nrf2* mRNA expression and CAT and Cu/ZnSOD enzyme activities. This increase in *Nrf2* is consistent with in vitro data showing that CA [65] and CA derivatives [66] exert their protective effect via the Nrf2 pathway. The results obtained with CA administration on antioxidant enzyme activities are slightly different from the effect observed with *A. borbonica* polyphenol-rich extract. Indeed, when compared to the UUO + Veh group, we observed a significant increase in CAT activity, and the increase in GPX activity was not significantly different. In addition, we did not observe a significant effect on carbonylated proteins. In fact, the observed effect on antioxidant enzyme activity with the polyphenol-rich extract from *A. borbonica* may result from the combination of the different polyphenols' effects. Thus, these discrepancies could be related to the administered CA dose, which is much higher than the CA concentration in the polyphenol-rich extract from *A. borbonica*.

To provide more evidence that polyphenols can exert their biological effects at the kidney level, we used the DESI imaging technique to visualize and provide evidence that CA, given by oral route, is rapidly present in the kidney, strongly suggesting bioavailability of CA in the kidney. Our data are consistent with the biodistribution study of Omar et al. [67] which used [3-^{14}C]trans-caffeic acid. However, we observed a low bioavailability (F = 0.4%) probably due to an important metabolic activity in the intestine and liver prior to reaching the main blood stream. The presence of the CA metabolite ferulic acid, produced by the action of catechol-O-methyl transferase, confirms this hypothesis as previously reported [68,69]. DESI-HR/MS imaging allowed us to visualize, for the first time, CA and FA in the renal cortex. Regardless of the quantity of CA that reached the kidney tissue, our data strongly suggests that CA is involved in the nephroprotective effect of the polyphenol-rich extract from *A. borbonica*.

5. Conclusions

The present study demonstrates, for the first time, that both polyphenol-rich extract from *A. borbonica* and CA, which is the predominant polyphenol, significantly improves, in a curative way, renal tubulointerstitial fibrosis in the UUO mouse model, especially via their antioxidant and anti-inflammatory properties. Further studies will be necessary to validate this antifibrotic effect on chronic models of renal disease, such as diabetic nephropathy. Notably, we cannot rule out that part of the observed nephroprotective effects of *A. borbonica* could be mediated by other polyphenols present in the plant extract, such as quercetin and kaempferol. Indeed, further investigations will be necessary to determine the individual and synergistic effects between the main polyphenols found in *A. borbonica*, to better understand this nephroprotective effect before considering clinical trials.

Supplementary Materials: The following are available online at https://www.mdpi.com/article/10.3390/biomedicines9040358/s1, Table S1: The known nephrotoxic molecules not detected by UPLC-HESI-Q-Orbitrap (Q-Exactive^{TM} Plus) in *A. borbonica* extract.

Author Contributions: B.V. and J.-L.B. conceived and designed the experiments; B.V., M.B., C.T., P.R., C.P., I.A.-A. and F.G. performed the experiments; B.V., P.R. and J.-L.B. analyzed the data; M.-P.G., C.M., O.M., N.D. and J.-L.B. contributed reagents/materials/analysis tools; writing—original draft, B.V. and J.-L.B.; writing—review and editing, B.V., M.-P.G., O.M., N.D. and J.-L.B. All authors have read and agreed to the published version of the manuscript.

Funding: This research was funded by European Regional Development Funds (FEDER RE0022527 ZEBRATOX, EU-Région Réunion-French State national counterpart), the University of La Réunion, the Institut National de la Santé et de la Recherche Médicale and the Reunion dotation funds Philancia. Bryan Veeren is a recipient of a fellowship from the Région Réunion.

Institutional Review Board Statement: All reported experiments were performed at the GIP-CYROI technological platform's animal facility (A974001), conducted in accordance with NIH guidelines for the care and use of laboratory animals, and were approved by the French authorities (APAFIS#7347-2016100314466830v5, approved on 4 September 2017).

Conflicts of Interest: The authors declare no conflict of interest.

References

1. Epstein, F.H.; Klahr, S.; Schreiner, G.; Ichikawa, I. The progression of renal disease. *N. Engl. J. Med.* **1988**, *318*, 1657–1666. [CrossRef] [PubMed]
2. Nath, K.A. Tubulointerstitial changes as a major determinant in the progression of renal damage. *Am. J. Kidney Dis.* **1992**, *20*, 1–17. [CrossRef]
3. Cohen, E. Fibrosis causes progressive kidney failure. *Med. Hypotheses* **1995**, *45*, 459–462. [CrossRef]
4. Nangaku, M. Mechanisms of tubulointerstitial injury in the kidney: Final common pathways to end-stage renal failure. *Intern. Med.* **2004**, *43*, 9–17. [CrossRef]
5. Hewitson, T.D. Renal tubulointerstitial fibrosis: Common but never simple. *Am. J. Physiol. Physiol.* **2009**, *296*, F1239–F1244. [CrossRef]
6. Liu, Y. Cellular and molecular mechanisms of renal fibrosis. *Nat. Rev. Nephrol.* **2011**, *7*, 684–696. [CrossRef] [PubMed]
7. Heart Outcomes Prevention Evaluation Study Investigators. Effects of ramipril on cardiovascular and microvascular outcomes in people with diabetes mellitus: Results of the HOPE study and MICRO-HOPE substudy. *Lancet* **2000**, *355*, 253–259. [CrossRef]
8. Pitt, B.; A Poole-Wilson, P.; Segal, R.; A Martinez, F.; Dickstein, K.; Camm, A.J.; A Konstam, M.; Riegger, G.; Klinger, G.H.; Neaton, J.; et al. Effect of losartan compared with captopril on mortality in patients with symptomatic heart failure: Randomised trial—the Losartan Heart Failure Survival Study ELITE II. *Lancet* **2000**, *355*, 1582–1587. [CrossRef]
9. Lewis, E.J.; Hunsicker, L.G.; Clarke, W.R.; Berl, T.; Pohl, M.A.; Lewis, J.B.; Ritz, E.; Atkins, R.C.; Rohde, R.; Raz, I. Renoprotective effect of the angiotensin-receptor antagonist irbesartan in patients with nephropathy due to type 2 diabetes. *N. Engl. J. Med.* **2001**, *345*, 851–860. [CrossRef] [PubMed]
10. Eckardt, K.-U.; Coresh, J.; Devuyst, O.; Johnson, R.J.; Köttgen, A.; Levey, A.S.; Levin, A. Evolving importance of kidney disease: From subspecialty to global health burden. *Lancet* **2013**, *382*, 158–169. [CrossRef]
11. Sridhar, V.S.; Rahman, H.U.; Cherney, D.Z. What have we learned about renal protection from the cardiovascular outcome trials and observational analyses with SGLT2 inhibitors? *Diabetes Obes. Metab.* **2020**, *22*, 55–68. [CrossRef]
12. Schernthaner, G.; Groop, P.; Kalra, P.A.; Ronco, C.; Taal, M.W. Sodium-glucose linked transporter-2 inhibitor renal outcome modification in type 2 diabetes: Evidence from studies in patients with high or low renal risk. *Diabetes Obes. Metab.* **2020**, *22*, 1024–1034. [CrossRef]
13. Hodrea, J.; Balogh, D.B.; Hosszu, A.; Lenart, L.; Besztercei, B.; Koszegi, S.; Sparding, N.; Genovese, F.; Wagner, L.J.; Szabo, A.J.; et al. Reduced O-GlcNAcylation and tubular hypoxia contribute to the antifibrotic effect of SGLT2 inhibitor dapagliflozin in the diabetic kidney. *Am. J. Physiol. Physiol.* **2020**, *318*, F1017–F1029. [CrossRef]
14. Allinovi, M.; De Chiara, L.; Angelotti, M.L.; Becherucci, F.; Romagnani, P. Anti-fibrotic treatments: A review of clinical evidence. *Matrix Biol.* **2018**, *68-69*, 333–354. [CrossRef]
15. Moreno, J.A.; Gomez-Guerrero, C.; Mas, S.; Sanz, A.B.; Lorenzo, O.; Ruiz-Ortega, M.; Opazo, L.; Mezzano, S.; Egido, J. Targeting inflammation in diabetic nephropathy: A tale of hope. *Expert Opin. Investig. Drugs* **2018**, *27*, 917–930. [CrossRef] [PubMed]
16. Lv, W.; Booz, G.W.; Fan, F.; Wang, Y.; Roman, R.J. Oxidative Stress and Renal Fibrosis: Recent Insights for the Development of Novel Therapeutic Strategies. *Front. Physiol.* **2018**, *9*, 105. [CrossRef]
17. Ow, C.P.C.; Ngo, J.P.; Ullah, M.; Hilliard, L.M.; Evans, R.G. Renal hypoxia in kidney disease: Cause or consequence? *Acta Physiol.* **2018**, *222*, e12999. [CrossRef] [PubMed]
18. Vanherweghem, J.-L.; Tielemans, C.; Abramowicz, D.; Depierreux, M.; Vanhaelen-Fastre, R.; Vanhaelen, M.; Dratwa, M.; Richard, C.; Vandervelde, D.; Verbeelen, D.; et al. Rapidly progressive interstitial renal fibrosis in young women: Association with slimming regimen including Chinese herbs. *Lancet* **1993**, *341*, 387–391. [CrossRef]
19. Jadot, I.I.; Declèves, A.-E.; Nortier, J.; Caron, N. An Integrated View of Aristolochic Acid Nephropathy: Update of the Literature. *Int. J. Mol. Sci.* **2017**, *18*, 297. [CrossRef] [PubMed]
20. Giraud-Techer, S.; Amedee, J.; Girard-Valenciennes, E.; Thomas, H.; Brillant, S.; Grondin, I.; Marodon, C.; Smadja, J. Plantes medi-cinales de la Réunion inscrites à la pharmacopée française. *Ethnopharmacologia* **2016**, *5*, 7–33.
21. Adsersen, A.; Adsersen, H. Plants from Réunion Island with alleged antihypertensive and diuretic effects—An experimental and ethnobotanical evaluation. *J. Ethnopharmacol.* **1997**, *58*, 189–206. [CrossRef]

22. Marimoutou, M.; Le Sage, F.; Smadja, J.; D'Hellencourt, C.L.; Gonthier, M.-P.; Silva, C.R.-D. Antioxidant polyphenol-rich extracts from the medicinal plants Antirhea borbonica, Doratoxylon apetalum and Gouania mauritiana protect 3T3-L1 preadipocytes against H2O2, TNFα and LPS inflammatory mediators by regulating the expression of superoxide dismutase and NF-κB genes. *J. Inflamm.* **2015**, *12*, 1–15. [CrossRef]
23. Fortin, H.; Vigor, C.; Dévéhat, F.L.-L.; Robin, V.; Le Bossé, B.; Boustie, J.; Amoros, M. In vitro antiviral activity of thirty-six plants from La Réunion Island. *Fitoter* **2002**, *73*, 346–350. [CrossRef]
24. LeDoux, A.; Cao, M.; Jansen, O.; Mamede, L.; Campos, P.-E.; Payet, B.; Clerc, P.; Grondin, I.; Girard-Valenciennes, E.; Hermann, T.; et al. Antiplasmodial, anti-chikungunya virus and antioxidant activities of 64 endemic plants from the Mascarene Islands. *Int. J. Antimicrob. Agents* **2018**, *52*, 622–628. [CrossRef]
25. Haddad, J.G.; Koishi, A.C.; Gaudry, A.; Dos Santos, C.N.D.; Viranaicken, W.; Desprès, P.; El Kalamouni, C. Doratoxylon apetalum, an Indigenous Medicinal Plant from Mascarene Islands, Is a Potent Inhibitor of Zika and Dengue Virus Infection in Human Cells. *Int. J. Mol. Sci.* **2019**, *20*, 2382. [CrossRef]
26. Lavergne, R. *Tisaneurs et Plantes Médicinales Indigènes à la Réunion*; Orphie: Livry Gargan, France, 2016; ISBN 979-10-298 0073-3.
27. Poullain, C.; Girard-Valenciennes, E.; Smadja, J. Plants from reunion island: Evaluation of their free radical scavenging and antioxidant activities. *J. Ethnopharmacol.* **2004**, *95*, 19–26. [CrossRef]
28. Taïlé, J.; Arcambal, A.; Clerc, P.; Gauvin-Bialecki, A.; Gonthier, M.-P. Medicinal Plant Polyphenols Attenuate Oxidative Stress and Improve Inflammatory and Vasoactive Markers in Cerebral Endothelial Cells during Hyperglycemic Condition. *Antioxidants* **2020**, *9*, 573. [CrossRef]
29. Delveaux, J.; Turpin, C.; Veeren, B.; Diotel, N.; Bravo, S.B.; Begue, F.; Álvarez, E.; Meilhac, O.; Bourdon, E.; Rondeau, P. Antirhea borbonica Aqueous Extract Protects Albumin and Erythrocytes from Glycoxidative Damages. *Antioxidants* **2020**, *9*, 415. [CrossRef] [PubMed]
30. Ghaddar, B.; Veeren, B.; Rondeau, P.; Bringart, M.; D'Hellencourt, C.L.; Meilhac, O.; Bascands, J.-L.; Diotel, N. Impaired brain homeostasis and neurogenesis in diet-induced overweight zebrafish: A preventive role from A. borbonica extract. *Sci. Rep.* **2020**, *10*, 1–17. [CrossRef]
31. Arcambal, A.; Taïlé, J.; Couret, D.; Planesse, C.; Veeren, B.; Diotel, N.; Gauvin-Bialecki, A.; Meilhac, O.; Gonthier, M. Protective Effects of Antioxidant Polyphenols against Hyperglycemia-Mediated Alterations in Cerebral Endothelial Cells and a Mouse Stroke Model. *Mol. Nutr. Food Res.* **2020**, *64*, e1900779. [CrossRef]
32. Veeren, B.; Ghaddar, B.; Bringart, M.; Khazaal, S.; Gonthier, M.-P.; Meilhac, O.; Diotel, N.; Bascands, J.-L. Phenolic Profile of Herbal Infusion and Polyphenol-Rich Extract from Leaves of the Medicinal Plant Antirhea borbonica: Toxicity Assay Determination in Zebrafish Embryos and Larvae. *Molecules* **2020**, *25*, 4482. [CrossRef]
33. Clifford, M.N.; Kerimi, A.; Williamson, G. Bioavailability and metabolism of chlorogenic acids (acyl-quinic acids) in hu-mans. *Compr. Rev. Food Sci. Food Saf.* **2020**, *19*, 1299–1352. [CrossRef] [PubMed]
34. Schramm, T.; Hester, Z.; Klinkert, I.; Both, J.P.; Heeren, R.M.; Brunelle, A.; Laprévote, O.; Desbenoit, N.; Robbe, M.F.; Stoeckli, M.; et al. imzML—A common data format for the flexible exchange and processing of mass spectrometry imaging data. *J. Proteom.* **2012**, *75*, 5106–5110. [CrossRef] [PubMed]
35. Källback, P.; Nilsson, A.; Shariatgorji, M.; Andrén, P.E. msIQuant–Quantitation Software for Mass Spectrometry Imaging Enabling Fast Access, Visualization, and Analysis of Large Data Sets. *Anal. Chem.* **2016**, *88*, 4346–4353. [CrossRef]
36. Schanstra, J.P.; Neau, E.; Drogoz, P.; Gomez, M.A.A.; Novoa, J.M.L.; Calise, D.; Pécher, C.; Bader, M.; Girolami, J.-P.; Bascands, J.-L. In vivo bradykinin B2 receptor activation reduces renal fibrosis. *J. Clin. Investig.* **2002**, *110*, 371–379. [CrossRef]
37. Singleton, V.L.; Rossi, J.A. Colorimetry of Total Phenolics with Phosphomolybdic-PhosphotungsticAcid Reagents. *Am. J. Enol. Vitic.* **1965**, *16*, 144–158.
38. Zhishen, J.; Mengcheng, T.; Jianming, W. The determination of flavonoid contents in mulberry and their scavenging effects on superoxide radicals. *Food Chem.* **1999**, *64*, 555–559. [CrossRef]
39. Klein, J.; Gonzalez, J.; Duchene, J.; Esposito, L.; Pradere, J.P.; Neau, E.; Delage, C.; Calise, D.; Ahluwalia, A.; Carayon, P.; et al. Delayed blockade of the kinin B1 receptor reduces renal inflammation and fibrosis in obstructive nephropathy. *FASEB J.* **2008**, *23*, 134–142. [CrossRef] [PubMed]
40. Rondeau, P.; Navarra, G.; Cacciabaudo, F.; Leone, M.; Bourdon, E.; Militello, V. Thermal aggregation of glycated bovine serum albumin. *Biochim. Biophys. Acta (BBA) Proteins Proteom.* **2010**, *1804*, 789–798. [CrossRef]
41. De Smet, P.A.G.M. Herbal remedies. *N. Engl. J. Med.* **2002**, *347*, 2046–2056. [CrossRef]
42. Colson, C.R.; De Broe, M.E. Kidney injury from alternative medicines. *Adv. Chronic Kidney Dis.* **2005**, *12*, 261–275. [CrossRef] [PubMed]
43. Yang, B.; Xie, Y.; Guo, M.; Rosner, M.H.; Yang, H.; Ronco, C. Nephrotoxicity and Chinese herbal medicine. *Clin. J. Am. Soc. Nephrol.* **2018**, *13*, 1605–1611. [CrossRef] [PubMed]
44. Bascands, J.-L.; Schanstra, J.P. Obstructive nephropathy: Insights from genetically engineered animals. *Kidney Int.* **2005**, *68*, 925–937. [CrossRef]
45. Eddy, A.A.; López-Guisa, J.M.; Okamura, D.M.; Yamaguchi, I. Investigating mechanisms of chronic kidney disease in mouse models. *Pediatr. Nephrol.* **2011**, *27*, 1233–1247. [CrossRef] [PubMed]

46. Kim, T.-W.; Kim, Y.-J.; Seo, C.-S.; Kim, H.-T.; Park, S.-R.; Lee, M.-Y.; Jung, J.-Y. Elsholtzia ciliata (Thunb.) Hylander attenuates renal inflammation and interstitial fibrosis via regulation of TGF-ß and Smad3 expression on unilateral ureteral obstruction rat model. *Phytomedicine* **2016**, *23*, 331–339. [CrossRef] [PubMed]
47. Hosseinian, S.; Bideskan, A.E.; Shafei, M.N.; Sadeghnia, H.R.; Soukhtanloo, M.; Shahraki, S.; Noshahr, Z.S.; Rad, A.K. Nigella sativa extract is a potent therapeutic agent for renal inflammation, apoptosis, and oxidative stress in a rat model of unilateral ureteral obstruction. *Phytother. Res.* **2018**, *32*, 2290–2298. [CrossRef]
48. Zhou, X.; Zhang, J.; Xu, C.; Wang, W. Curcumin ameliorates renal fibrosis by inhibiting local fibroblast proliferation and extracellular matrix deposition. *J. Pharmacol. Sci.* **2014**, *126*, 344–350. [CrossRef]
49. Chen, H.; Chen, C.-M.; Guan, S.-S.; Chiang, C.-K.; Wu, C.-T.; Liu, S.-H. The antifibrotic and anti-inflammatory effects of icariin on the kidney in a unilateral ureteral obstruction mouse model. *Phytomedicine* **2019**, *59*, 152917. [CrossRef]
50. Liu, S.; Zhao, M.; Zhou, Y.; Wang, C.; Yuan, Y.; Li, L.; Bresette, W.; Chen, Y.; Cheng, J.; Lu, Y.; et al. Resveratrol exerts dose-dependent anti-fibrotic or pro-fibrotic effects in kidneys: A potential risk to individuals with impaired kidney function. *Phytomedicine* **2019**, *57*, 223–235. [CrossRef]
51. Liu, X.; Sun, N.; Mo, N.; Lu, S.; Song, E.; Ren, C.; Li, Z. Quercetin inhibits kidney fibrosis and the epithelial to mesenchymal transition of the renal tubular system involving suppression of the Sonic Hedgehog signaling pathway. *Food Funct.* **2019**, *10*, 3782–3797. [CrossRef]
52. Wang, Y.; Wang, B.; Du, F.; Su, X.; Sun, G.; Zhou, G.; Bian, X.; Liu, N. Epigallocatechin-3-gallate attenuates unilateral ureteral obstruction-induced renal interstitial fibrosis in mice. *J. Histochem. Cytochem.* **2014**, *63*, 270–279. [CrossRef]
53. Scalbert, A.; Johnson, I.T.; Saltmarsh, M. Polyphenols: Antioxidants and beyond. *Am. J. Clin. Nutr.* **2005**, *81*, 215S–217S. [CrossRef]
54. Wakabayashi, N.; Slocum, S.L.; Skoko, J.J.; Shin, S.; Kensler, T.W. When NRF2 talks, who's listening? *Antioxid. Redox Signal.* **2010**, *13*, 1649–1663. [CrossRef]
55. Bocci, V.; Valacchi, G. Nrf2 activation as target to implement therapeutic treatments. *Front. Chem.* **2015**, *3*, 4. [CrossRef] [PubMed]
56. Zecher, M.; Guichard, C.; Velásquez, M.J.; Figueroa, G.; Rodrigo, R. Implications of oxidative stress in the pathophysiology of obstructive uropathy. *Urol. Res.* **2008**, *37*, 19–26. [CrossRef] [PubMed]
57. Aminzadeh, M.A.; Nicholas, S.B.; Norris, K.C.; Vaziri, N.D. Role of impaired Nrf2 activation in the pathogenesis of oxidative stress and inflammation in chronic tubulo-interstitial nephropathy. *Nephrol. Dial. Transplant.* **2013**, *28*, 2038–2045. [CrossRef] [PubMed]
58. Zhou, Y.; Jiang, Z.; Lu, H.; Xu, Z.; Tong, R.; Shi, J.; Jia, G. Recent Advances of Natural Polyphenols Activators for Keap1-Nrf2 Signaling Pathway. *Chem. Biodivers.* **2019**, *16*, e1900400. [CrossRef]
59. Wang, W.; Wang, X.; Zhang, X.-S.; Liang, C.-Z. Cryptotanshinone Attenuates Oxidative Stress and Inflammation through the Regulation of Nrf-2 and NF-κB in Mice with Unilateral Ureteral Obstruction. *Basic Clin. Pharmacol. Toxicol.* **2018**, *123*, 714–720. [CrossRef]
60. Wang, Y.; Wang, B.; Du, F.; Su, X.; Sun, G.; Zhou, G.; Bian, X.; Liu, N. Epigallocatechin-3-Gallate Attenuates Oxidative Stress and Inflammation in Obstructive Nephropathy via NF-κB and Nrf2/HO-1 Signalling Pathway Regulation. *Basic Clin. Pharmacol. Toxicol.* **2015**, *117*, 164–172. [CrossRef] [PubMed]
61. Dendooven, A.; Ishola, D.A., Jr.; Nguyen, T.Q.; Van Der Giezen, D.M.; Kok, R.J.; Goldschmeding, R.; Joles, J.A. Oxidative stress in obstructive nephropathy. *Int. J. Exp. Pathol.* **2010**, *92*, 202–210. [CrossRef]
62. Damasceno, S.S.; Dantas, B.B.; Ribeiro-Filho, J.; Araújo, D.A.M.; Da Costa, J.G.M. Chemical Properties of Caffeic and Ferulic Acids in Biological System: Implications in Cancer Therapy. A Review. *Curr. Pharm. Des.* **2017**, *23*, 3015–3023. [CrossRef]
63. Chuang, S.-T.; Kuo, Y.-H.; Su, M.-J. Antifibrotic effects of KS370G, a caffeamide derivative, in renal ischemia-reperfusion injured mice and renal tubular epithelial cells. *Sci. Rep.* **2014**, *4*, srep05814. [CrossRef] [PubMed]
64. Chuang, S.-T.; Kuo, Y.-H.; Su, M.-J. KS370G, a caffeamide derivative, attenuates unilateral ureteral obstruction-induced renal fibrosis by the reduction of inflammation and oxidative stress in mice. *Eur. J. Pharmacol.* **2015**, *750*, 1–7. [CrossRef] [PubMed]
65. Pan, Y.; Deng, Z.-Y.; Chen, X.; Zhang, B.; Fan, Y.; Li, H. Synergistic antioxidant effects of phenolic acids and carotenes on H2O2-induced H9c2 cells: Role of cell membrane transporters. *Food Chem.* **2021**, *341*, 128000. [CrossRef]
66. Peng, X.; Wu, G.; Zhao, A.; Huang, K.; Chai, L.; Natarajan, B.; Yang, S.; Chen, H.; Lin, C. Synthesis of novel caffeic acid derivatives and their protective effect against hydrogen peroxide induced oxidative stress via Nrf2 pathway. *Life Sci.* **2020**, *247*, 117439. [CrossRef]
67. Omar, M.H.; Mullen, W.; Stalmach, A.; Auger, C.; Rouanet, J.-M.; Teissedre, P.-L.; Caldwell, S.T.; Hartley, R.C.; Crozier, A. Absorption, disposition, metabolism, and excretion of [3-(14)C]caffeic acid in rats. *J. Agric. Food Chem.* **2012**, *60*, 5205–5214. [CrossRef]
68. Crozier, A.; Del Rio, D.; Clifford, M.N. Bioavailability of dietary flavonoids and phenolic compounds. *Mol. Asp. Med.* **2010**, *31*, 446–467. [CrossRef] [PubMed]
69. Stalmach, A.; Williamson, G.; Clifford, M.N. Dietary hydroxycinnamates and their bioavailability. In *Flavonoids and Related Compounds: Bioavailability and Function*; CRC Press: Boca Raton, FL, USA, 2012; Volume 30, Available online: https://research.monash.edu/en/publications/dietary-hydroxycinnamates-and-their-bioavailability (accessed on 30 March 2021).

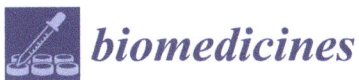

Article

Curcumin and Radiotherapy Exert Synergistic Anti-Glioma Effect In Vitro

Vasiliki Zoi [1], Vasiliki Galani [2], Evrysthenis Vartholomatos [1], Natalia Zacharopoulou [1], Eftichia Tsoumeleka [1], Georgios Gkizas [1], Georgios Bozios [3], Pericles Tsekeris [4], Ieremias Chousidis [5], Ioannis Leonardos [5], Andreas G. Tzakos [6], Athanasios P. Kyritsis [1] and George A. Alexiou [1,*]

[1] Neurosurgical Institute, University of Ioannina, 45500 Ioannina, Greece; vasozoi95@gmail.com (V.Z.); eyrys.varth@gmail.com (E.V.); nataliezacharop13@gmail.com (N.Z.); eutuxiatsoum@gmail.com (E.T.); geogkizas@hotmail.com (G.G.); thkyrits@uoi.gr (A.P.K.)
[2] Department of Anatomy Histology-Embryology, School of Medicine, University of Ioannina, 45110 Ioannina, Greece; vgalani@uoi.gr
[3] Department of Medical Physics, University of Ioannina, 45110 Ioannina, Greece; gbozios@uhi.gr
[4] Department of Radiation Oncology, University of Ioannina, 45110 Ioannina, Greece; ptsekeri@uoi.gr
[5] Zoology Laboratory, Department of Biological Application and Technology, University of Ioannina, 45110 Ioannina, Greece; i.chousidis@uoi.gr (I.C.); ileonard@uoi.gr (I.L.)
[6] Department of Chemistry, Section of Organic Chemistry and Biochemistry, University of Ioannina, 45110 Ioannina, Greece; atzakos@uoi.gr
* Correspondence: galexiou@uoi.gr

Abstract: Curcumin, a bioactive polyphenol, is known to have anticancer properties. In this study, the effectiveness of curcumin pretreatment as a strategy for radio-sensitizing glioblastoma cell lines was explored. For this, U87 and T98 cells were treated with curcumin, exposed to 2 Gy or 4 Gy of irradiation, and the combined effect was compared to the antiproliferative effect of each agent when given individually. Cell viability and proliferation were evaluated with the trypan blue exclusion assay and the 3-(4,5-dimethylthiazol-2-yl)-2,5-diphenyltetrazolium bromide (MTT) assay. The synergistic effects of the combination treatment were analyzed with CompuSyn software. To examine how the co-treatment affected different phases of cell-cycle progression, a cell-cycle analysis via flow cytometry was performed. Treatment with curcumin and radiation significantly reduced cell viability in both U87 and T98 cell lines. The combination treatment arrested both cell lines at the G2/M phase to a higher extent than radiation or curcumin treatment alone. The synergistic effect of curcumin when combined with temozolomide resulted in increased tumor cell death. Our results demonstrate for the first time that low doses of curcumin and irradiation exhibit a strong synergistic anti-proliferative effect on glioblastoma cells in vitro. Therefore, this combination may represent an innovative and promising strategy for the treatment of glioblastoma, and further studies are needed to fully understand the molecular mechanism underlying this effect.

Keywords: curcumin; glioblastoma cells; radiation

1. Introduction

Glioblastoma is the most common and severe Central Nervous System (CNS) tumor accounting for 45.6% of all primary malignant brain tumors [1,2]. In spite of intensive clinical investigation, the median survival remains around 15 months, and recurrence is almost universal since the tumor shows significant resistance to all existing therapeutic approaches. Many chemotherapeutic agents have been used against glioblastoma, including temozolomide (TMZ) [3,4]. Chemoresistance has been proven to be a major challenge for successful treatment, and several different chemoresistance mechanisms have been investigated and reported [5]. The presence of the blood–brain barrier and the highly aggressive infiltration of glioblastoma into the surrounding tissues has, so far, surmounted effective treatment [6].

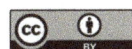

Multiple epidemiological studies have explored the role of natural compounds in the development, progress, and survival of cancer cells [7]. Several natural compounds known for their antioxidant and chemotherapeutic properties, including soy, curcumin, resveratrol, and retinoids, have been reported as possible therapeutic compounds against glioblastoma [8]. Curcumin is a polyphenol extracted from the rhizome of the plant Curcuma longa, which belongs to the *Zingiberaceae* family. Curcumin has exhibited a prominent role in the treatment of several health conditions, including metabolic syndrome, inflammatory disorders, neurodegenerative diseases, as well as different types of cancer [9–11]. The majority of the antitumor effects of curcumin include cell-cycle arrest, inhibition of oncogenes, and increased apoptosis of cancer cells [12]. Curcumin's antiproliferative effects are related to different molecular pathways, such as nuclear factor κB (NF-κB), Akt, and Wnt/β-catenin [13–15]. NF-κB is overexpressed in GBM and its deregulation is related to increased tumor growth and cell cycle progression, whereas the Wnt/β-catenin pathway affects cell proliferation, differentiation, and tumorigenesis [16,17]. Curcumin has been found to suppress the NF-κB signaling pathway through the blockage of constitutive Akt and JNK activation [18]. Moreover, through inhibition of the WNT/β-catenin pathway, curcumin can decrease the expression of cyclin D1 and thus inhibit the development and proliferation of gliomas [19]. The utilization of curcumin is associated with certain limitations, including poor oral bioavailability, rapid metabolism, and elimination. However, the use of nanotechnology drug-delivery systems such as liposomes, nanoparticles, or micelles can help overcome those limitations [20]. Furthermore, the molecular weight of curcumin is 368.38 Daltons and is thus able to cross the blood–brain barrier (BBB) (Figure 1).

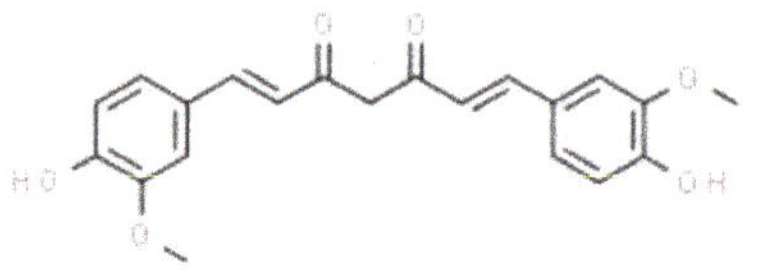

Figure 1. Structure of curcumin. It was drawn using ChemSpider, an online free chemical structure database.

Since radiotherapy belongs to the standard treatment of glioblastoma (GBM) patients, the radiosensitizing potential of curcumin in human glioma cells is worth taking note of. Both the dose range and timing of curcumin administration when combined with irradiation are important. The present study was designed to investigate the antitumor effects of curcumin, both alone and in combination with radiotherapy in glioblastoma cell lines. Our results suggest that the co-treatment of curcumin and radiation resulted in significant cell death and inhibited cell growth more effectively than either single treatment did.

2. Results

2.1. Curcumin Inhibits Glioblastoma Cell Proliferation

The effects of curcumin on cell viability are displayed in Figure 2. The IC50 value of curcumin determined after 72 h post-treatment was 10 µM in U87 cells and 13 µM in T98. To further delineate the effects of curcumin on cell proliferation, Crystal Violet staining of U87 and T98 cells was performed and photos using phase-contrast microscopy were taken at 72 h. Increasing concentrations of curcumin induced changes in the morphology of both cell lines, including cell shrinkage, indicating cell death (Figure 3a,b).

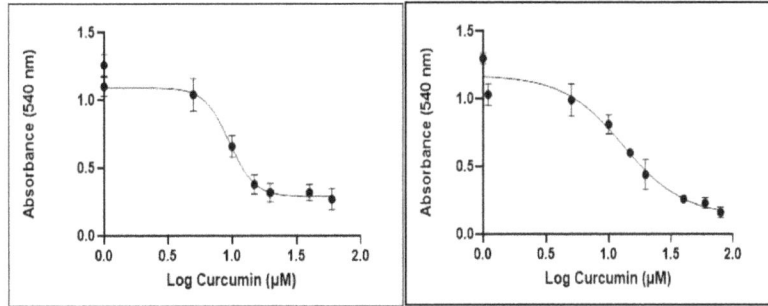

Figure 2. Cytotoxic effect of curcumin on glioblastoma cell lines U87 and T98 at 72 h. Values shown are the means and standard deviations from three independent experiments and are normalized to non-treated cells ($p < 0.05$ vs. control). The IC50 values were determined using the non-linear regression analysis model of GraphPad Prism Version 8.

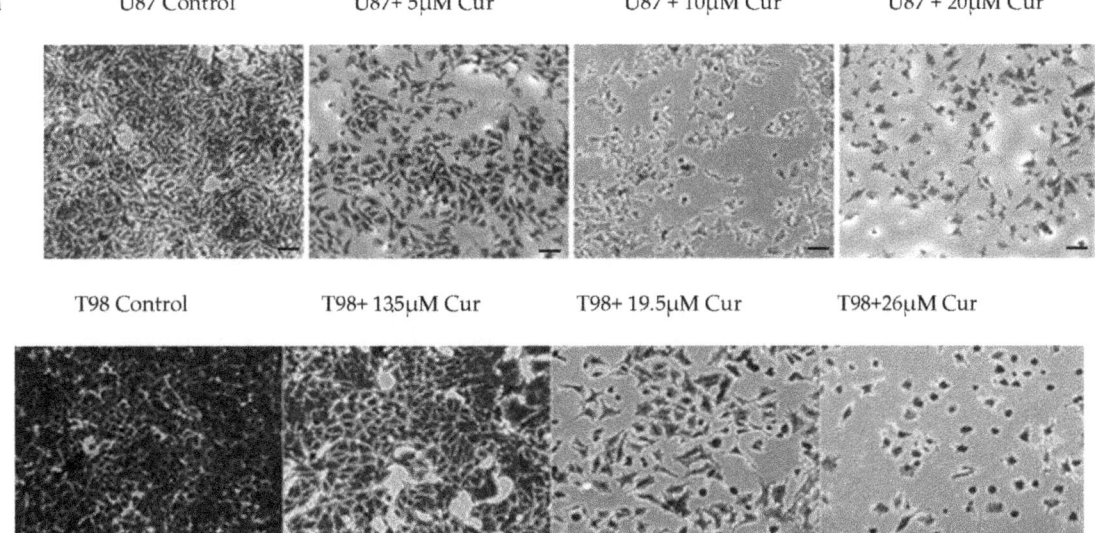

Figure 3. Morphological changes in U87 (**a**) and T98 (**b**) cell populations after treatment with crystal violet staining (0.2% Crystal Violet) (Scale bars = 50 μm). Images were recorded at 10× magnification. Cells were seeded in 6-well plates and 24 h later exposed to increasing curcumin concentrations. Crystal violet solution was added 48 h later and the cells were incubated at room temperature for 2–3 min. The excess crystal violet was removed, and plates were washed twice and left overnight to dry.

2.2. Combinatorial Effect of Curcumin and Irradiation on Glioblastoma Cells

Curcumin was used in concentrations ranging from 5–25 μM and 3.25–26 μM in U87 and T98 cells, respectively, whereas radiation was given in doses of 2 or 4 Gy. The effect of curcumin in combination with radiation is summarized in Tables 1 and 2. In U87 cells, curcumin and radiation exerted synergism in the majority of tested combinations, and the highest synergy was monitored when curcumin was given at its IC50 value, namely 10 μM. In T98 cells, the highest levels of synergy were observed at higher curcumin concentrations, particularly at 26 μM, possibly due to the resistance of those cells to both chemotherapy and radiotherapy. Overall, curcumin and radiation exhibited a strong synergistic relationship in both cell lines, except for some mild antagonistic behavior at lower curcumin concentrations, 5 µM in U87 cells and 6.5 and 13 µM in T98 cells, possibly due to the inability of curcumin to sensitize glioblastoma cells to the cytotoxic effects of irradiation at lower doses; however, further studies are needed.

Table 1. Assessment of combinatorial effect of curcumin and radiation in U87 cells. CI was determined by CompuSyn software.

Curcumin (µM)	Radiation (Gy)	Effect	CI	Conclusion
5	2	0.3	1.14445	Antagonism
10	2	0.85	0.6062	Synergism
15	2	0.86	0.84063	Synergism
20	2	0.92	0.84358	Synergism
25	2	0.94	0.91683	Synergism
5	4	0.43	1.15321	Antagonism
10	4	0.86	0.66052	Synergism
15	4	0.89	0.81149	Synergism
20	4	0.92	0.89425	Synergism
25	4	0.93	1.02773	Antagonism

Table 2. Assessment of combinatorial effect of curcumin and radiation in T98 cells. CI was determined by CompuSyn software.

Curcumin (µM)	Radiation (Gy)	Effect	CI	Conclusion
3.25	2	0.44	0.74507	Synergism
6.5	2	0.49	1.0575	Antagonism
13	2	0.74	1.04795	Antagonism
26	2	0.95	0.71409	Synergism
3.25	4	0.48	0.97007	Synergism
6.5	4	0.53	1.22819	Antagonism
13	4	0.68	1.38199	Antagonism
26	4	0.97	0.53544	Synergism

The graphical representation of the combinatorial effect of curcumin and radiation is also presented via the dose–effect curves and combination index plots that were created using CompuSyn software for U87 (Figure 4a,b) and T98 (Figure 5a,b) cell lines.

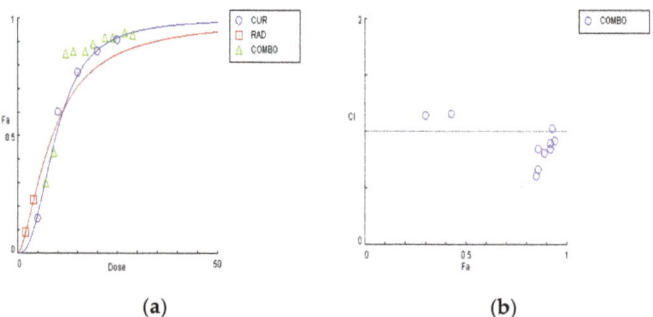

(a) (b)

Figure 4. Graphical presentations obtained from the CompuSyn Report for the curcumin and radiation combination in U87 cells. (**a**) Dose–effect curve; (**b**) combination index plot.

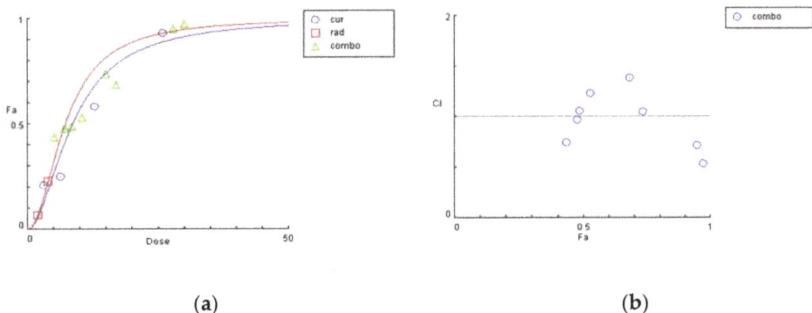

Figure 5. Graphical presentations obtained from the CompuSyn Report for the curcumin and radiation combination in T98 cells. (**a**) Dose–effect curve; (**b**) combination index plot.

For each drug combination, CompuSyn calculates the dose–reduction index where DRI > 1 and <1 indicate a favorable and not favorable dose–reduction, respectively, and DRI = 1 indicates no dose-reduction. As seen in Figure 6, in both U87 (a) and T98 (b) cell lines, most combinations of curcumin and radiation show a favorable dose–reduction (DRI > 1).

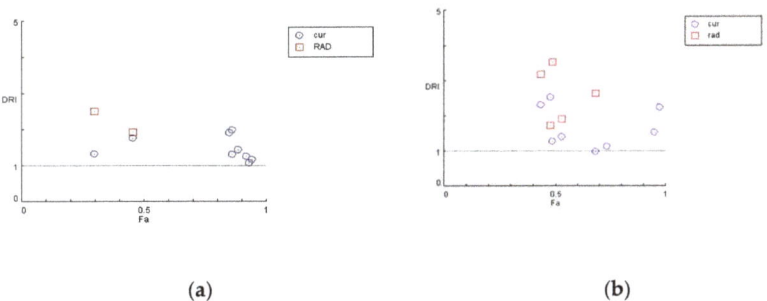

Figure 6. Dose reduction plots for the combination of curcumin and radiation at different experimental points for U87 (**a**) and T98 (**b**) cells. DRI >1 shows favorable dose reduction of both factors.

2.3. Curcumin Enhanced the Radiation-Induced G2/M Arrest in Glioblastoma Cells

Since curcumin treatment in combination with radiation brought significant cytotoxicity in both U87 and T98 cell lines, it was important to explore how the combination treatment affected different phases of cell-cycle progression. For this, a flow cytometric analysis with DNA staining dye, propidium iodide (PI), was performed. Cell cultures were treated with increasing curcumin concentrations for 72 h. At 72 h, the cells were stained with PI and the DNA content was calculated. Curcumin induced both an S and G2/M arrest in U87 and T98 cells when given alone. Interestingly, when cells were treated with IC50 and 2IC50 concentrations of curcumin along with 2 Gy of radiation, the percentage distribution of the cells in the G2/M phase was enhanced considerably in both U87 (Figure 7) and T98 (Figure 8) cell lines. Specifically, when U87 cells were treated with 20 µM of curcumin, followed by 2 Gy, the percentage distribution of cells in the G2/M phase (20.9%) was enhanced significantly compared to treatment with curcumin alone (13%), under the same conditions. Accordingly, in the T98 cell line, treatment with 15 µM of curcumin, followed by 2 Gy, resulted in a higher-percentage distribution of cells in the G2/M phase (22.9%) compared to treatment with 15 µM of curcumin alone (13.5%). Since the G2/M phase is arrested as a result of DNA damage, the above results show that curcumin may be enhancing the damaging effects of radiation.

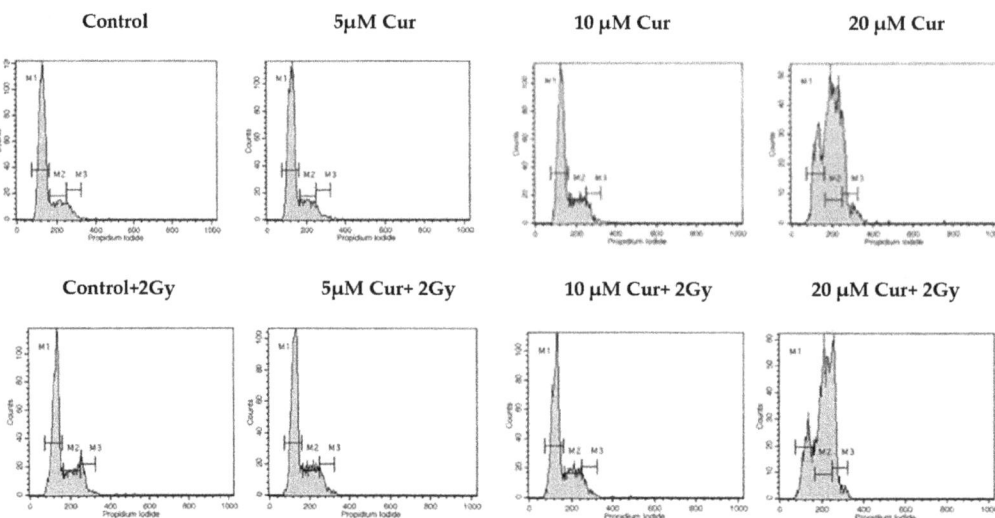

Figure 7. Histogram representation of cell-cycle distribution in U87 cells after treatment with increasing curcumin concentrations. Cells (10^4) were seeded in 24-well plates and after 24 h were exposed to different curcumin concentrations; 2 h later, the plates were irradiated with 2 Gy. After 72 h, the cells were stained with propidium iodide and the DNA content was observed.

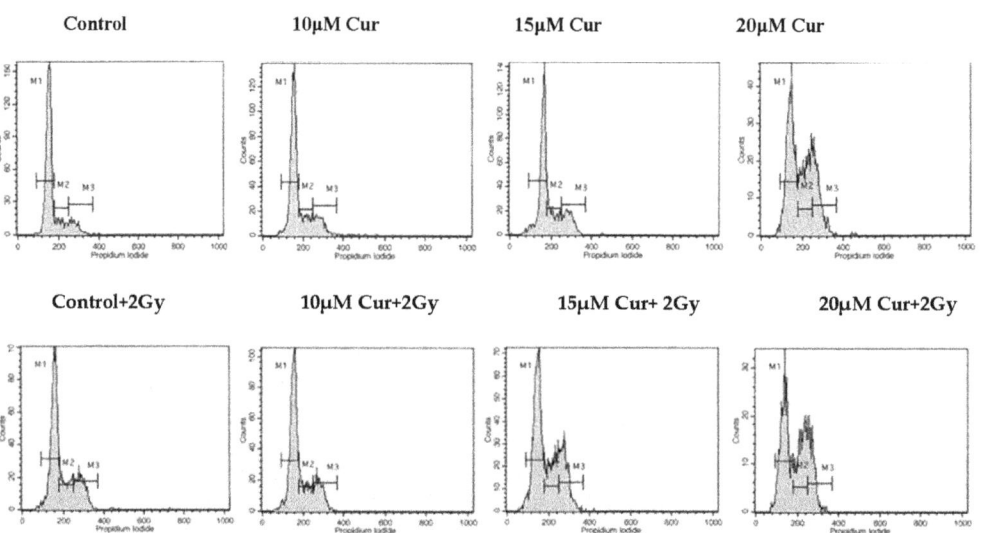

Figure 8. Histogram representation of cell-cycle distribution in T98 cells after treatment with increasing curcumin concentrations. Following the same procedure, the cells were stained with propidium iodide at 72 h, and the DNA content was observed. Curcumin and radiation co-treatment induced G2/M arrest in glioblastoma cells.

2.4. Curcumin and Temozolomide Exhibited Synergistic Anti-Proliferative Effect on Glioma Cells

Prior to examining the synergistic effect of curcumin and TMZ, the effective dose for TMZ was determined using the trypan blue exclusion assay. U87 cells were seeded at a density of 10^4 in 24-well plates for 24 h and then increased concentrations of TMZ were added. The cells were incubated for another 72 h, at the end of which trypan blue dye was added to each well. The cytotoxic effects of TMZ in U87 cells are presented in Figure 9.

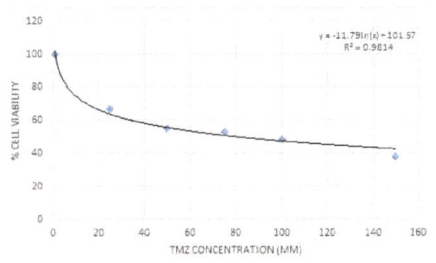

Figure 9. Cytotoxic effect of temozolomide on glioblastoma cell line U87. The IC50 value for temozolomide was calculated at 80 µM with an $R^2 = 0.9814$.

To determine the synergism or antagonism of the combination of curcumin and TMZ in U87 cells, curcumin was used in concentrations ranging from 2.5–20 µM in U87, whereas TMZ was given in concentrations ranging 20–160 µM. Combination therapy was carried out in a constant ratio of 1:8 (cur: TMZ) and the combined effect of the two drugs factors was compared with the effect of each drug separately. Curcumin and TMZ exerted strong synergism in all combinations tested (CI < 1). When given together, a favorable dose–reduction effect was observed for both drugs on each combination point (DRI > 1). Both combination index and dose–reduction plots were developed with the use of CompuSyn (Figure 10a,b).

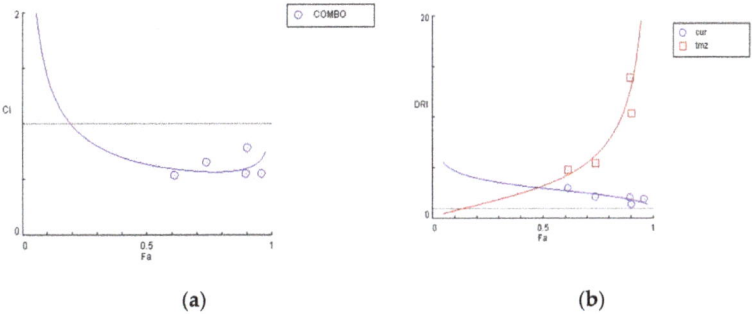

Figure 10. Graphical presentations obtained from the CompuSyn Report for the curcumin and temozolomide combination in U87 cells. (**a**) Combination index plot; (**b**) dose–reduction plot.

2.5. Zebrafish Lethal Concentration Determination

The toxic effect is induced in a concentration-dependent manner. The mortality rate rises as the concentration increases. The lethal dose was LC50 = 20.89 µM, while LC25 and LC75 were 18.50 µM and 23.35 µM, respectively (Figure 11).

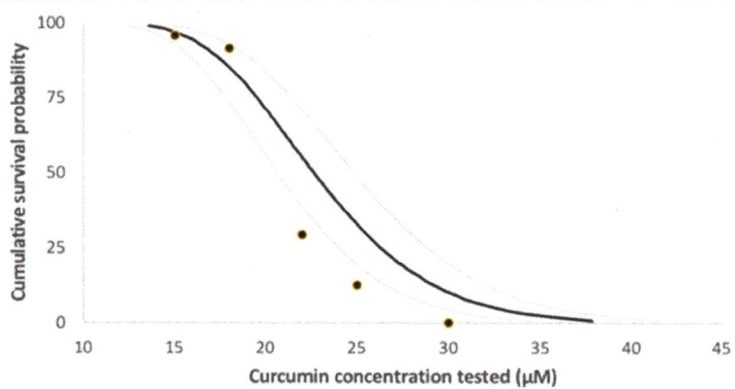

Figure 11. Lethal concentration determination.

3. Discussion

Glioblastoma is the most common and severe tumor of the CNS [1]. Many chemotherapeutic agents have been used against glioblastoma, including TMZ [3]. Radiotherapy and chemotherapy belong to the standard treatment of glioblastoma, following surgical resection. However, both chemo and radio resistance has been proven to be a major challenge for the successful treatment of GBM. Researchers have attempted to identify novel radiosensitizers to achieve better clinical outcomes, including natural compounds.

Curcumin is a natural polyphenol that has been used for centuries in traditional Chinese medicine in the treatment of allergies, infections, and respiratory disorders [21]. In recent years, phytochemicals, and curcumin in particular, have garnered the interest of various scientific groups worldwide in both experimental and pre-clinical studies for their effects on different types of cancer.

The present study unveiled that curcumin and radiation are an effective combination in the treatment of glioblastoma in vitro. Curcumin inhibited cell proliferation and caused cell-cycle arrest in both U87 and T98 cell lines. When combined with irradiation, its anti-proliferative properties were further enhanced. In a zebrafish model, no significant mortality was observed at curcumin concentrations of up to 18 μM. Since glioblastoma is difficult to cure via neurosurgery or radiotherapy alone, the combination of curcumin and radiation could be a potentially promising treatment.

In previous studies, curcumin was investigated for its ability to exert radiosensitizing effects on different cell types. Kunwar et al. examined the cellular uptake of curcumin and confirmed that cancer cells (T cell lymphoma of murine origin and human breast cancer cells) showed relatively higher uptake of curcumin compared to normal cells (mouse spleen lymphocytes and fibroblast cells) [22]. Zanotto-Filho et al. studied the effects of curcumin on the proliferation of glioblastoma cell lines in vitro, as well as in a preclinical model in vivo. Curcumin induced cell death and inhibited proliferation in four glioma cell lines at IC50 values of 19–28 μM. In vivo, curcumin reduced the size of intracranially growing tumors in rats, and showed no evidence of toxicity in healthy tissues [23]. Rodriguez et al. investigated the role of curcumin in glioblastoma, analyzing 19 in vitro and 5 in vivo studies. All studies showed that curcumin induced cell death through a series of molecular mechanisms, including the activation of apoptotic pathways via caspace-3, p21, and p53 [24].

Glioblastoma remains the most aggressive and invasive primary brain tumor in adults. Current treatment includes surgical excision, followed by chemotherapy and radiotherapy. However, despite aggressive treatment, recurrence is, in most cases, an inevitable event [2]. The presence of BBB is an important contributor to glioblastoma's resistance to chemotherapy. Curcumin, theoretically, can pass through the BBB thanks to its relatively low molecular weight and lipophilic nature. [10] In most of the studies carried out on animals, curcumin was given orally [25]. In rats, after oral administration of a 2 g/kg dose, curcumin reached a maximum serum concentration of 1.35 µg/mL. However, when the same dosage was given to humans, the serum levels of curcumin were extremely low (0.006 µg/mL). When mice were given 50 mg/kg curcumin orally, a brain concentration lower than the limit of detection was observed 60 or 120 min after administration [26]. On the contrary, when mice were fed for up to 4 months with curcumin (2.5–10 mg/day orally), they showed 0.5 µg/g brain tissue [27]. The low absorption rate, its rapid metabolism, and systemic elimination are the major obstacles that deprive it from reaching satisfactory serum levels in humans after oral administration [28].

Radiotherapy remains a significant part of every treatment regimen against glioblastoma; however, it has not been used thoroughly in the investigation of combination treatments for GBM [29]. The possible photosensitizing effects of curcumin in vitro have been explored by a few scientific groups. Jamali et al. examined the effects of curcumin on the DKMG human cell line when given along with photodynamic therapy (radiation dose 60 J/cm^2). Their results indicated an important curcumin dose–reduction in cell proliferation [30]. Back in 2007, Dhandapani et al. investigated the combinatorial effects of curcumin and irradiation. In their study, they treated two glioma lines, U87 and T98, with curcumin alone at a concentration of 25 µM, irradiation alone (5 Gy using a 137Cs γ-cell-40 Exactor), and their combination. They observed that a synergistic effect of curcumin and radiation existed in both cell lines as a result of the inhibition of anti-apoptotic gene expression and that the maximum% cell death induced by this combination was about 60% [18]. In the present study, we found that the combination of curcumin and radiation can induce cytotoxicity of up to 94% and 95% for the U87 and T98 cell lines, respectively, accompanied by favorable dose–reduction. For glioblastoma, based on the pivotal phase 3 trial published in 2005, standard treatment includes 60 Gy in 2 Gy fractions delivered over 6 weeks [31]. Taking into account our previous studies as well, and in order to follow the standard treatment protocol, we used a dose of 2 or 4 Gy using X-rays generated by a linac 6 MV accelerator [32]. The most prominent synergistic effect was observed when curcumin was given at its IC50 value, namely 10 µM for the U87 cell line, whereas for the more-resistant T98 cell line, a concentration of 26 µM demonstrated the highest synergy. In both cases, 2 Gy of radiation was enough to produce that strong synergetic effect.

Curcumin induced G2/M cell-cycle arrest when given alone and that effect was further enhanced when combined with irradiation. Back in 2015, Zhang et al. investigated the potent radiosensitizing effects of curcumin on U87 human glioma cells in vivo. Nude mice bearing subcutaneous U87 xenografts were treated with 50 mg/kg of curcumin and exposed to 5 Gy of irradiation. The results showed that curcumin significantly increased the radiosensitivity of U87 cells in vivo via the enhancement of the dual-specificity phosphatase (DUSP-2) pathway [33]. The exact molecular mechanisms of the radiosensitization of curcumin are still under investigation; however, it is known that drugs that produce G2/M arrest are potent radiosensitizers [34]. When DNA damage occurs, the DNA damage checkpoint is activated, which involves ATM kinase activation and autophosphorylation at Ser1981. This can induce cell-cycle arrest to delay the proliferation of cancer cells. Since cells in the G2/M phase are more sensitive to radiation, this arrest may be a significant strategy in the treatment of GBM [35]. In the present study, we found that low doses of curcumin increased the number of cells undergoing G2/M phase arrest. Radiation can also result in G2/M phase arrest and apoptosis. Thus, the addition of curcumin can induce the transformation of cancer cells into a more radiosensitive status. When curcumin was given with TMZ, which is the major chemotherapeutic drug against glioblastoma, a synergistic anti-proliferative effect on both cell lines was also observed. Therefore, a combinatorial treatment using curcumin, temozolomide, and low doses of irradiation may be a promising future treatment option. Preclinical studies on the combinatorial effect of curcumin and radiation are depicted in Table 3. Our current results show that a combinatorial treatment using curcumin and low doses of irradiation may be a promising future treatment option.

Table 3. Studies on the combinatorial effect of curcumin and irradiation in different in vitro and in vivo GBM models.

In Vitro/In Vivo Effect	Mechanism of Action	Dosing/Duration	References
Synergetic effect of curcumin when combined with irradiation on T98G and U87MG cells in vitro	Decrease in anti-apoptotic gene expression	25 µM curcumin 6 h prior to 5 Gy radiation	Dhandapani et al. [18]
In vivo radiosensitization of U87 glioma xenografts in vivo	Upregulation of DUSP-2, inhibition of ERK/JNK phosphorylation	50 mg/kg plus irradiation (5 Gy) every 2 days, curcumin 2 h prior to radiation	Zhang et al. [33]
No radiosensitizing effect of curcumin on cell viability in U251 glioma cells in vitro	Clonogenic cell survival in U251 cells is reduced after 96 h at doses exceeding 5 µM	5 µM curcumin 72 h prior to 1–6 Gy single dose	Sminia et al. [36]

The present study has several limitations. Following repeated intake of curcumin in humans, plasma concentrations have been found to be relatively low, peaking at approximately 2 µM [37]. Mean intratumoral concentrations of curcumin have been reported to be around 0.15 µM after oral administration [38]. Novel technical approaches to increase the bioavailability of curcumin include encapsulation in nanoparticles, the use of liquid micelles, or micronized powder [39,40]. Moreover, evaluating the combined effects of curcumin and radiation 72 h after treatment may be preliminary and may require additional experiments, including a colony-forming assay where the effects on cell viability are more prominently observed 10–14 days after treatment [41]. Therefore, further experiments are needed to fully determine the degree of synergy between curcumin and radiation in glioblastoma cells. Although we found synergistic anti-cancer effects of curcumin and radiation in cultured glioblastoma cells lines, the mechanistic details of glioblastoma growth, proliferation, invasion, and metastasis in animal or human brains are much more complex. For this reason, a complete understanding of the mechanism of the combined effects of curcumin and radiotherapy will require additional experiments in animals to optimize the therapeutic strategy prior to clinical use.

In summary, this study is the first to demonstrate that co-treatment of curcumin and radiation shows higher inhibitory effects compared to their individual administration and results in a more prominent G2/M arrest in the cell cycle of both U87 and T98 cell lines. Given that glioblastoma is a highly heterogenic tumor, difficult to treat, with the additional obstacle of the presence of BBB, the need for novel and effective anti-cancer drugs is a clearly unmet clinical need. Further studies will be necessary to better understand the synergistic effects of curcumin and radiation on glioblastoma treatment and validate our results in glioma xenograft models prior to clinical trials.

4. Materials and Methods

4.1. Cell Lines and Treatment Conditions

The human glioma cell line T98 was obtained from ATCC (Manassas, VA, USA), whereas the U87 cell line was obtained from Dr W.K. Alfred Yung (Department of Neuro-Oncology, M.D. Anderson Cancer Center, Houston, TX, USA). Both cell lines were cultured in Dulbecco's Modified Eagle's Medium (Gibco BRL, Life Technologies, Grand Island, NY, USA), supplemented with 10% fetal bovine serum (FBS) and 1% penicillin–streptomycin (Gibco BRL). Both cell lines were incubated in a humidified atmosphere regulated at 5% CO_2 and 37 °C. The medium was changed every three days. Curcumin (Sigma Aldrich, St. Louis, MO, USA) was dissolved in DMSO to a stock concentration of 36 mM and stored at 4 °C. TMZ (Sigma Aldrich, St. Louis, MO, USA) was dissolved in dimethyl sulfoxide and stored as a stock solution of 103 mM at 4 °C. Before each experiment, curcumin and TMZ were diluted from their stock solution to the final concentration with a culture medium.

Less than 1% of DMSO was present in the final volumes of each experiment. Cultures of glioma cells were treated with curcumin alone or in combination with radiotherapy or TMZ.

4.2. Viability Assay

Cultures of human glioma cells were treated with curcumin in concentrations of 1, 5, 10, 15, 20, 40, and 60 µM for the U87 cell line and in concentrations of 1, 5, 10, 15, 20, 40, 60, and 80 µM for the T98 cell line. Cell viability was evaluated by the Trypan Blue exclusion assay and the 3-(4,5-dimethylthiazol-2-yl)-2,5-diphenyltetrazolium bromide (MTT, Sigma Aldrich, St. Louis, MO, USA assay) [42,43]. A Trypan Blue exclusion assay was performed in 24-well plates where 10,000 cells were seeded, and after 24 h, were exposed to increasing concentrations of curcumin. Cell viability was determined at 72 h with the use of a phase-contrast microscope. For the MTT assay, 2000 cells were seeded in 96-well plates, and after 24 h, were exposed to the same increasing concentrations of curcumin. The cells were incubated for another 72 h and then MTT was added. The amount of MTT-formazan was determined at 570 nm. Both methods were performed three times, and the results presented are the mean of the three. Changes in cell proliferation were also continuously determined with the use of a phase-contrast microscope. The Trypan Blue assay was also used for the determination of cell viability in U87 cells after exposure to increased concentrations of TMZ.

4.3. Crystal Violet Assay

The crystal violet assay was used to further determine cell proliferation in both U87 and T98 cell lines after exposure to increased curcumin concentrations. Cells were seeded at a density of 10^5 per well in 6-well plates, and after 24 h, curcumin was added in increased concentrations. The cells were incubated for 48 h, washed twice with phosphate-buffered saline (PBS), and further incubated for 2–3 min with the Crystal Violet Solution 0.2% (0.2 g Crystal Violet Powder, MERCK, MA, USA) in 80 mL of ddH_2O and 20 mL Methanol. Plates were then rinsed with running water and left overnight to dry. Pictures of each well-plate were taken the next day with the use of phase-contrast microscopy.

4.4. Flow Cytometric Analysis of DNA Cell Cycle

Cells (10^4) were treated with increased concentrations of curcumin alone or in combination with radiation. Untreated cells were used as a negative control with 1% of DMSO. At least three independent experiments were performed, and all samples were run in triplicates. Flow cytometric analysis was performed on day 5. For the DNA cell cycle, cells were treated with trypsin, centrifuged, washed well with PBS, and then incubated with PI-working solution (50 µg/mL PI, 20 mg/mL RNase A, and 0.1% Triton X-100) for 20 min at 37 °C in the dark. With the use of a flow cytometer (FACScalibur, BD Biosciences, San Jose, CA, USA), the PI fluorescence of 10,000 individual nuclei was determined. Using the CellQuest software program (BD Biosciences, CA, USA), the fractions of cells in G0/G1, S, G2/M, and sub-G0/G1 phases were analyzed [44].

4.5. Combination Treatment with Curcumin and Radiation

Cells (10^4) were treated with different concentrations of either curcumin alone or a combination of curcumin and radiation. U87 and T98 cells were cultured in 24-well plates and after 24 h were treated with curcumin. After 2 h, the cells were irradiated at 2 Gy or 4 Gy as described previously [32]. Cell viability was determined using the Trypan Blue exclusion assay at 72 h. The combinatorial effect of curcumin and radiation was evaluated using the combination index method of Chou and Talalay [45]. Curcumin was used in concentrations of 5, 10, 15, 20, and 25 µM for the U87 cell line and at concentrations of 3.25, 6.5, 13, and 26 µM for the T98 cell line. Two different doses of irradiation were used in both cell lines, 2 and 4 Gy. A total of 10 and 8 different combinations with three replicates per condition were used for the U87 and T98 cell lines, respectively. The affected fraction of cells after treatment with curcumin alone, irradiation alone, or different combinations of those two was calculated, and the dose–effect curves were generated. The Combination Index (CI) was determined using CompuSyn software (Compusyn, Inc., Paramus, NJ, USA). The CI value determines the effect of the combination treatment. A CI < 1 is considered synergistic, a CI = 1 is considered additive, and a CI > 1 is considered antagonistic [46].

4.6. Combination Treatment with Curcumin and Temozolomide

Cells (10^4) were treated with different concentrations of either curcumin, TMZ, or a combination of curcumin and TMZ. U87 cells were cultured in 24-well plates and after 24 h were treated with curcumin and/or TMZ, and the Trypan Blue exclusion assay was performed at 72 h. The dose–effect parameters of each drug alone or in different combinations were automatically determined from the median-effect equation created by CompuSyn software.

4.7. Zebrafish

4.7.1. Zebrafish Housing and Husbandry

Adult zebrafish of the wild-type strain (AB) were maintained in a colony room in a recirculated system at 28 ± 1 °C, pH 6.5–7.5, conductivity 500 ± 50 µS cm^{-1} with a 14-h light/10-h dark photoperiod (lights on at 8:00 a.m.). Feeding of the fish was performed twice per day following common practices (with zebrafish feed). Sexually mature zebrafish (at least three-months old) were used for spawning. Embryos were collected and pooled into a standard zebrafish E3 culture medium (5 mmol/L NaCl, 0.33 mmol/L CaCl$_2$, 0.33 mmol/L MgSO$_4$·7H$_2$O, and 0.17 mmol/L KCl).

4.7.2. Zebrafish Toxicity Testing

The collection of zebrafish embryos was performed at the beginning of the 14 h light cycle following the mating procedure that took place overnight. After the inspection of the embryos, those that were unfertilized or showed significant malformation were removed, and the dechorionation process followed at 24 hpf. The dechorionated embryos were placed in 24-well culture plates (2 embryos per well, 1.5 mL of solution per well) and each experiment was performed in triplicate. In the current study, five different concentrations of curcumin were tested (0, 15, 18, 22, 25, 30 µM). In total, 248 embryos were studied, of which 48 per each concentration were in the control group.

4.7.3. Lethal Concentration (LC50) Determination

Preliminary tests were performed in order to evaluate the full 0–100% range of mortality. The concentration range was 15 to 30 µM. Toxicity assays (LC50 calculation) and confidence intervals (LC25 and LC75) were determined based on cumulative mortality at the end of the experiment.

4.8. Statistical Analysis

All results are presented as the mean ± standard deviation (SD). IC50 values were determined with the use of GraphPad Prism software (v. 8.0.0, San Diego, California USA, Trial Version) through regression analysis. Multiple comparisons of groups were analyzed using two-way ANOVA with the post hoc Tukey test. Parameters of LC50 were assessed using a regression Probit analysis (the chi-square test, Pearson goodness of fit test, and 95% confidence interval). Analyses were performed using SPSS statistical software v26 (IBM Corp., Armonk, NY, USA). Differences were considered significant at p-values < 0.05.

Author Contributions: Conceptualization, G.A.A., A.P.K., and V.G.; methodology, V.Z., G.G., E.V., P.T., I.L. and A.G.T., data curation, V.Z., E.V., N.Z., E.T., I.C. and G.B., writing—original draft preparation, V.Z., V.G., G.A.A., A.P.K., I.L., A.G.T. and P.T.; writing—review and editing, G.A.A., A.P.K., V.G., A.G.T. and I.L.; visualization, supervision, G.A.A., A.P.K. and V.G. All authors have read and agreed to the published version of the manuscript.

Funding: This research received no external funding.

Institutional Review Board Statement: Not applicable.

Informed Consent Statement: Not applicable.

Conflicts of Interest: The authors declare no conflict of interest.

References

1. Klinger, N.V.; Mittal, S. Therapeutic Potential of Curcumin for the Treatment of Brain Tumors. *Oxid. Med. Cell Longev.* **2016**, *5*, 1–14. [CrossRef]
2. Weathers, S.P.; Gilbert, M.R. Advances in treating glioblastoma. *Prime Rep.* **2014**, *6*, 46. [CrossRef]
3. Tsamis, K.I.; Alexiou, G.A.; Vartholomatos, E.; Kyritsis, A.P. Combination treatment for glioblastoma cells with tumor necrosis factor-related apoptosis-inducing ligand and oncolytic adenovirus delta-24. *Cancer Investig.* **2013**, *31*, 630–638. [CrossRef]
4. Kyritsis, A.P.; Levin, V.A. An algorithm for chemotherapy treatment of recurrent glioma patients after temozolomide failure in the general oncology setting. *Cancer Chemother. Pharmacol.* **2011**, *67*, 971–983. [CrossRef]
5. Alexiou, G.A.; Goussia, A.; Voulgaris, S.; Fotopoulos, A.D.; Fotakopoulos, G.; Ntoulia, A.; Zikou, A.; Tsekeris, P.; Argyropoulou, M.I.; Kyritsis, A.P. Prognostic significance of MRP5 immunohistochemical expression in glioblastoma. *Cancer Chemother. Pharmacol.* **2012**, *69*, 1387–1391. [CrossRef]
6. Sandberg, C.J.; Altschuler, G.; Jeong, J.; Strømme, K.K.; Stangeland, B.; Murrell, W.; Grasmo-Wendler, U.H.; Myklebost, O.; Helseth, E.; Vik-Mo, E.O. Comparison of glioma stem cells to neural stem cells from the adult human brain identifies dysregulated Wnt- signaling and a fingerprint associated with clinical outcome. *Exp. Cell Res.* **2013**, *319*, 2230–2243. [CrossRef]
7. Sarkar, F.H.; Li, Y.; Wang, Z.; Kong, D. Cellular signaling perturbation by natural products. *Cell. Signal.* **2009**, *21*, 1541–1547. [CrossRef]
8. Kyritsis, A.P.; Bondy, M.L.; Levin, V.A. Modulation of glioma risk and progression by dietary nutrients and antiinflammatory agents. *Nutr. Cancer.* **2011**, *63*, 174–184. [CrossRef]
9. Yung, W.K.; Kyritsis, A.P.; Gleason, M.J.; Levin, V.A. Treatment of recurrent malignant gliomas with highdose 13-cis-retinoic acid. *Clin. Cancer Res.* **1996**, *2*, 1931–1935.
10. Unlu, A.; Nayir, E.; Kalenderoglu, M.D.; Kirca, O.; Ozdogan, M. Curcumin (Turmeric) and cancer. *J. BUON* **2016**, *21*, 1050–1060.
11. Hewlings, S.J.; Kalman, D.S. Curcumin: A Review of Its' Effects on Human Health. *Foods* **2017**, *22*, 92. [CrossRef]
12. Zoi, V.; Galani, V.; Lianos, G.D.; Voulgaris, S.; Kyritsis, A.P.; Alexiou, G.A. The Role of Curcumin in Cancer Treatment. *Biomedicines* **2021**, *9*, 1086. [CrossRef]
13. Mukhopadhyay, A.; Banerjee, S.; Stafford, L.J.; Xia, C.; Liu, M.; Aggarwal, B.B. Curcumin-induced suppression of cell proliferation correlates with down-regulation of cyclin D1 expression and CDK4-mediated retinoblastoma protein phosphorylation. *Oncogene* **2002**, *21*, 8852–8861. [CrossRef]
14. Hatanpaa, K.J.; Burma, S.; Zhao, D.; Habib, A.A. Epidermal growth factor receptor in glioma: Signal transduction, neuropathology, imaging, and radioresistance. *Neoplasia* **2010**, *12*, 675–684. [CrossRef]
15. Elamin, M.H.; Shinwari, Z.; Hendrayani, S.F.; Al-Hindi, H.; Al-Shail, E.; Khafaga, Y.; Aboussekhra, A. Curcumin inhibits the Sonic Hedgehog signaling pathway and triggers apoptosis in medulloblastoma cells. *Mol. Carcinog.* **2010**, *49*, 302–314. [CrossRef]
16. Nagai, S.; Washiyama, K.; Kurimoto, M.; Takaku, A.; Endo, S.; Kumanishi, T. Aberrant nuclear factor-κB activity and its participation in the growth of human malignant astrocytoma. *J. Neurosurg.* **2002**, *96*, 909–917. [CrossRef]
17. Bahrami, A.; Amerizadeh, F.; ShahidSales, S.; Khazaei, M.; Ghayour-Mobarhan, M.; Sadeghnia, H.R.; Avan, A. Therapeutic potential of targeting Wnt/β-catenin pathway in treatment of colorectal cancer: Rational and progress. *J. Cell. Biochem.* **2017**, *118*, 1979–1983. [CrossRef]
18. Dhandapani, K.M.; Mahesh, V.B.; Brann, D.W. Curcumin suppresses growth and chemoresistance of human glioblastoma cells via AP-1 and NFκB transcription factors. *J. Neurochem.* **2007**, *102*, 522–538. [CrossRef]
19. He, M.; Li, Y.; Zhang, L.; Li, L.; Shen, Y.; Lin, L.; Zheng, W.; Chen, L.; Bian, X.; Ng, H.K.; et al. Curcumin suppresses cell proliferation through inhibition of the Wnt/β-catenin signaling pathway in medulloblastoma. *Oncol. Rep.* **2014**, *32*, 173–180. [CrossRef]
20. Mirzaei, H.; Khoi, M.J.M.; Azizi, M.; Goodarzi, M. Can curcumin and its analogs be a new treatment option in cancer therapy? *Cancer Gene Ther.* **2016**, *23*, 410. [CrossRef]
21. Ammon, H.P.; Wahl, M.A. Pharmacology of Curcuma longa. *Planta Med.* **1991**, *57*, 1–7. [CrossRef]
22. Kunwar, A.; Barik, A.; Mishra, B.; Rathinasamy, K.; Pandey, R.; Priyadarsini, K.I. Quantitative cellular uptake, localization and cytotoxicity of curcumin in normal and tumor cells. *Biochim. Biophys. Acta Gen. Subj.* **2008**, *1780*, 673–679. [CrossRef]
23. Zanotto-Filho, A.; Braganhol, E.; Edelweiss, M.I.; Behr, G.A.; Zanin, R.; Schröder, R.; Simões-Pires, A.; Battastini, A.M.; Moreira, J.C. The curry spice curcumin selectively inhibits cancer cells growth in vitro and in preclinical model of glioblastoma. *J. Nutr. Biochem.* **2012**, *23*, 591–601. [CrossRef]
24. Rodriguez, G.A.; Shah, A.H.; Gersey, Z.C.; Shah, S.S.; Bregy, A.; Komotar, R.J.; Graham, R.M. Investigating the therapeutic role and molecular biology of curcumin as a treatment for glioblastoma. *Ther. Adv. Med. Oncol.* **2016**, *8*, 248–260. [CrossRef]
25. Prasad, S.; Tyagi, A.K.; Aggarwal, B.B. Recent developments in delivery, bioavailability, absorption and metabolism of curcumin: The golden pigment from golden spice. *Cancer Res. Treat.* **2014**, *46*, 2–18. [CrossRef]

26. Schiborr, C.; Eckert, G.P.; Rimbach, G.; Frank, J. A validated method for the quantification of curcumin in plasma and brain tissue by fast narrow-bore high-performance liquid chromatography with fluorescence detection. *Anal. Bioanal. Chem.* **2010**, *5*, 1917–1925. [CrossRef]
27. Begum, A.N.; Jones, M.R.; Lim, G.P.; Morihara, T.; Kim, P.; Heath, D.D.; Rock, C.L.; Pruitt, M.A.; Yang, F.; Hudspeth, B.; et al. Curcumin structure-function, bioavailability, and efficacy in models of neuroinflammation and Alzheimer's disease. *J. Pharmacol. Exp. Ther.* **2008**, *1*, 196–208. [CrossRef] [PubMed]
28. Jamwal, R. Bioavailable curcumin formulations: A review of pharmacokinetic studies in healthy volunteers. *J. Integr. Med.* **2018**, *16*, 367–374. [CrossRef]
29. Levin, V.; Maor, M.; Thall, P.; Yung, W.; Bruner, J.; Sawaya, R.; Kyritsis, A.; Leeds, N.; Woo, S.; Rodríguez, L.; et al. Phase II study of accelerated fractionation radiation therapy with carboplatin followed by vincristine chemotherapy for the treatment of glioblastoma multiforme. *Int. J. Radiat. Oncol. Biol. Phys.* **1995**, *30*, 357–364. [CrossRef]
30. Jamali, Z.; Hejazi, S.M.; Ebrahimi, S.M.; Moradi-Sardareh, H.; Paknejad, M. Effects of LED-Based photodynamic therapy using red and blue lights, with natural hydrophobic photosensitizers on human glioma cell line. *Photodiagn. Photodyn. Ther.* **2018**, *21*, 50–54. [CrossRef]
31. Stupp, R.; Mason, W.P.; van den Bent, M.J.; Weller, M.; Fisher, B.; Taphoorn, M.J.; Belanger, K.; Brandes, A.A.; Marosi, C.; Bogdahn, U.; et al. Radiotherapy plus concomitant and adjuvant temozolomide for glioblastoma. *N. Engl. J. Med.* **2005**, *352*, 987–996. [CrossRef] [PubMed]
32. Alexiou, G.; Vartholomatos, E.; Tsamis, K.I.; Peponi, E.; Markopoulos, G.; Papathanasopoulou, V.; Tasiou, I.; Ragos, V.; Tsekeris, P.; Kyritsis, A.; et al. Combination treatment for glioblastoma with temozolomide, DFMO and radiation. *J. BUON* **2019**, *24*, 397–404.
33. Zhang, L.; Ding, X.; Huang, J.; Jiang, C.; Cao, B.; Qian, Y.; Cheng, C.; Dai, M.; Guo, X.; Shao, J. In vivo Radiosensitization of human glioma U87 cells induced by upregulated expression of DUSP-2 after treatment with curcumin. *Curr. Signal Transd. Ther.* **2015**, *10*, 119–125. [CrossRef]
34. Wang, Y.; Yang, L.; Zhang, J.; Zhou, M.; Shen, L.; Deng, W.; Liang, L.; Hu, R.; Yang, W.; Yao, Y.; et al. Radiosensitization by irinotecan is attributed to G2/M phase arrest, followed by enhanced apoptosis, probably through the ATM/Chk/Cdc25C/Cdc2 pathway in p53-mutant colorectal cancer cells. *Int. J. Oncol.* **2018**, *53*, 1667–1680. [PubMed]
35. Pawlik, T.M.; Keyomarsi, K. Role of cell cycle in mediating sensitivity to radiotherapy. *Int. J. Radiat. Oncol. Biol. Phys.* **2004**, *59*, 928–942. [CrossRef]
36. Sminia, P.; van den Berg, J.; van Kootwijk, A.; Hageman, E.; Slotman, B.J.; Verbakel, W. Experimental and clinical studies on radiation and curcumin in human glioma. *J. Cancer Res. Clin. Oncol.* **2021**, *147*, 403–409. [CrossRef]
37. Cheng, A.L.; Hsu, C.H.; Lin, J.K.; Hsu, M.M.; Ho, Y.F.; Shen, T.S.; Ko, J.Y.; Lin, J.T.; Lin, B.R.; Ming-Shiang, W.; et al. Phase I clinical trial of curcumin, a chemopreventive agent, in patients with high-risk or pre-malignant lesions. *Anticancer Res.* **2001**, *21*, 2895–2900.
38. Dutzmann, S.; Schiborr, C.; Kocher, A.; Pilatus, U.; Hattingen, E.; Weissenberger, J.; Gesler, F.; Quick-Weller, J.; Franz, K.; Seifert, V.; et al. Intratumoral concentrations and effects of orally administered micellar Curcuminoids in Glioblastoma patients. *Nutr. Cancer* **2016**, *68*, 943–948. [CrossRef]
39. Schiborr, C.; Kocher, A.; Behnam, D.; Jandasek, J.; Toelstede, S.; Frank, J. The oral bioavailability of curcumin from micronized powder and liquid micelles is significantly increased in healthy humans and differs between sexes. *Mol. Nutr. Food Res.* **2014**, *58*, 516–527. [CrossRef]
40. Kanai, M.; Imaizumi, A.; Otsuka, Y.; Sasaki, H.; Hashiguchi, M.; Tsujiko, K.; Matsumoto, S.; Ishiguro, H.; Chiba, T. Dose-escalation and pharmacokinetic study of nanoparticle curcumin, a potential anticancer agent with improved bioavailability, in healthy human volunteers. *Cancer Chemother. Pharmacol.* **2012**, *69*, 65–70. [CrossRef]
41. Franken, N.A.; Rodermond, H.M.; Stap, J.; Haveman, J.; van Bree, C. Clonogenic assay of cells in vitro. *Nat. Protoc.* **2006**, *1*, 2315–2319. [CrossRef] [PubMed]
42. Kastamoulas, M.; Chondrogiannis, G.; Kanavaros, P.; Vartholomatos, G.; Bai, M.; Briasoulis, E.; Arvanitis, D.; Galani, V. Cytokine effects on cell survival and death of A549 lung carcinoma cells. *Cytokine* **2013**, *61*, 816–825. [CrossRef] [PubMed]
43. Alexiou, G.A.; Tsamis, K.I.; Vartholomatos, E.; Peponi, E.; Tzima, E.; Tasiou, I.; Lykoudis, E.; Tsekeris, P.; Kyritsis, A.P. Combination treatment of TRAIL, DFMO and radiation for malignant glioma cells. *J. Neuro-Oncol.* **2015**, *123*, 217–224. [CrossRef] [PubMed]
44. Chondrogiannis, G.; Kastamoulas, M.; Kanavaros, P.; Vartholomatos, G.; Bai, M.; Baltogiannis, D.; Sofikitis, N.; Arvanitis, D.; Galani, V. Cytokine Effects on Cell Viability and Death of Prostate Carcinoma Cells. *BioMed Res. Int.* **2014**, *5*, 1–16. [CrossRef]
45. Chou, T.C. Theoretical Basis, Experimental Design, and Computerized Simulation of Synergism and Antagonism in Drug Combination Studies. *Pharmacol. Rev.* **2006**, *58*, 621–681. [CrossRef]
46. Chou, T.C. Drug Combination Studies and Their Synergy Quantification Using the Chou-Talalay Method. *Cancer Res.* **2010**, *70*, 440–446. [CrossRef] [PubMed]

MDPI
St. Alban-Anlage 66
4052 Basel
Switzerland
Tel. +41 61 683 77 34
Fax +41 61 302 89 18
www.mdpi.com

Biomedicines Editorial Office
E-mail: biomedicines@mdpi.com
www.mdpi.com/journal/biomedicines

www.ingramcontent.com/pod-product-compliance
Lightning Source LLC
LaVergne TN
LVHW070044120526
838202LV00101B/426